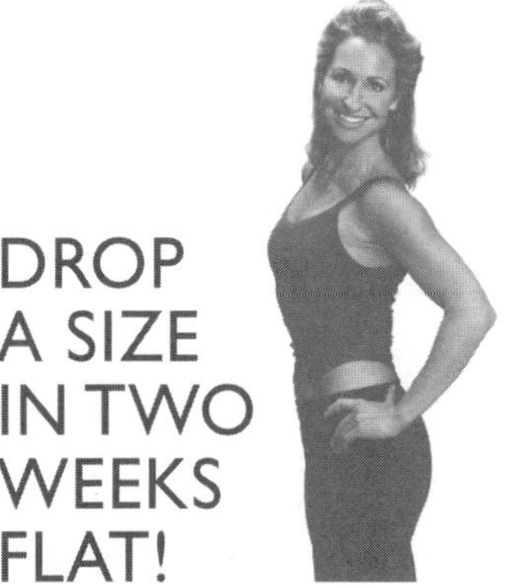
DROP
A SIZE
IN TWO
WEEKS
FLAT!

JOANNA HALL

with Sam Murphy

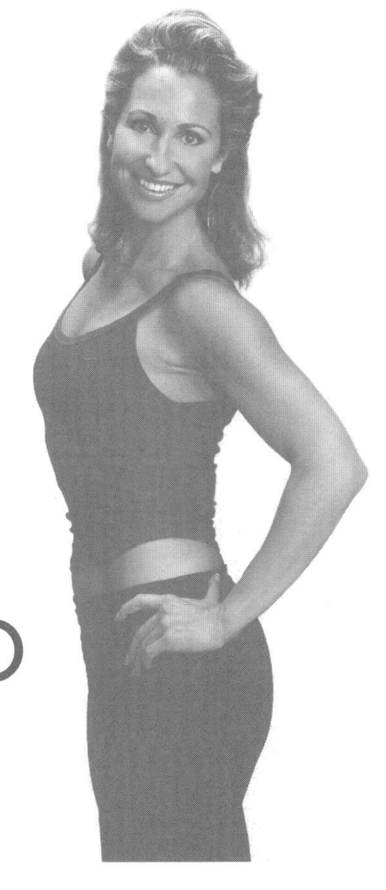

FOLLOW JOANNA'S STARCH CURFEW® PLAN AND LOSE FAT FAST

DROP A SIZE IN TWO WEEKS FLAT!

BARNES & NOBLE

NEW YORK

This edition published by Barnes & Noble Publishing Inc.,
by arrangement with HarperThorsons
an Imprint of HarperCollins*Publishers*

2005 Barnes & Noble Books

M 10 9 8 7 6 5 4 3 2 1

ISBN 0 7607 7787 X

Photography by Robin Matthews

Printed and bound in Thailand by
Imago

CONTENTS

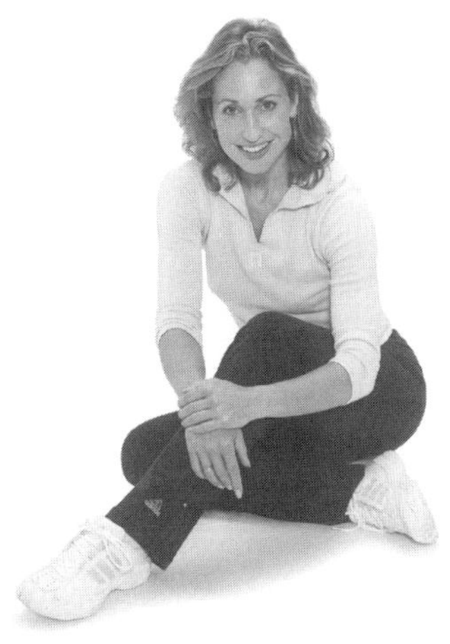

INTRODUCTION

How many times have you been on a diet? Less than five times? Ten times? More than 10? Or are you always on a diet? If dieting is a routine part of your life, you're not alone—6 out of 10 women are actively trying to lose weight at any one time, and there are literally hundreds of different diet plans, pills, and potions out there, all promising stunning weight loss results with minimum fuss and effort. The sad truth is that 95 percent of these weight loss efforts are unsuccessful in the long term. Yet despite all the previous failed attempts, you read about the latest quick-fix approach and think to yourself "yes, *this* time it's going to work"—only to find it's just another, albeit heavily disguised, version of the "No Air" diet.

The No Air diet! Well, think what happens when you hold your breath for as long as possible. As soon as you can't hold it any longer, you gasp in as much air as possible to make up for what you've been deprived of. It's exactly the same with dieting and getting fit—I have seen it so many times with clients. Instead of taking moderate, steady action, we dive in headfirst and embrace a totally unrealistic lifestyle, only to find we go off the rails a week later. Quite simply, the No Air diet doesn't work because it is unsustainable.

Here's a typical example …

MONDAY 136lb—v. bad. But not for long—I'm on my fab new diet!

Felt really psyched up when I woke up. Had black coffee for breakfast, a low cal soup for lunch and a low-calorie pre-packed slim meal in the evening. Didn't go out after work, what's the point if I can't have a few drinks? Went to bed stomach rumbling, but feeling incredibly virtuous.

TUESDAY 135lb—better. Had 1 cigarette (bad—but didn't inhale).

I was exhausted today—hardly slept thanks to my rumbling tummy. Black coffee for breakfast again, a plum mid-morning, and a low cal soup with a rice cake for lunch—tasted like styrofoam. Succumbed to a cigarette at lunchtime just to stop myself pigging out. Feeling pretty irritable by the afternoon. Had a couple of lettuce leaves for dinner and went to bed feeling curiously close to murdering someone.

WEDNESDAY 133lb—good. Succumbed to 8 cigarettes, 1 bottle of wine, 2 chocolate bars, a burger and fries—disastrous.

Oh dear! It was all going so well. I got through the morning on a couple of cigarettes with several large mugs of black coffee. Felt slightly spaced out and people at work were giving me a wide berth—I thought it was because I was a little irritable, but then Kate told me my breath reeked of coffee, yuck! Treated myself to two rice cakes with my low cal soup today, seeing as the weight seems to be falling off but then, about 4pm, I heard the candy machine calling me.

Before I knew it I'd scoffed two chocolate bars. So disillusioned was I that I stopped off at the burger joint on the way home from work (well, I'd blown it for today, so I thought I might as well start again tomorrow). And since the liquor store was next door, I bought a bottle of Chardonnay to wash it down.

THURSDAY 135lb—v. bad. No cigarettes—good.

I feel so guilty—can't believe I did that. Today I made up for the damage. Again, black coffee for breakfast, a slim shake for lunch and low cal soup for dinner (no rice cake). Went to bed feeling back in control but still annoyed with myself for yesterday's pig out.

FRIDAY 135lb—v. bad. Had 25 cigarettes, 6 gin and tonics and a pizza—v.v.bad.

Can't believe the pounds haven't dropped off after I was so good yesterday—life's so unfair. Went out after work and meant to ask for mineral water but it came out as G and T, and since I'd got through the day on rice cakes and diet coke, the alcohol hit an empty stomach and had me reeling. I felt better after the second one, but then, well, I don't remember much after that.

SATURDAY 136lb—v. bad.

Woke up clutching a half-eaten cold slice of pizza. Ow, my head hurts, but I'm meeting friends for lunch today—no chance of dieting there, and I'm going to the movies tonight, and can't possibly get through the movie without a large popcorn and a bag of chocolate-covered raisins. Ah well, Monday is less than 48 hours away and that's always a good day to start ...

Depressingly familiar, huh? Well, the good news is that this book is about helping you break free from the weight loss spiral and achieving a slimmer, healthier body that you can maintain for life. While the 14-day plan is low in calories, it is *not* a No Air diet. It's nutritionally sound, it's varied and it won't leave you hungry. But best of all it *does* work—as our volunteers found out when they took part in our trials. Follow the 14-day *Get a Grip* plan in section one, and you'll be slipping into a smaller size in no time. But wait! It's all very well fitting into size 10 jeans or a hip-hugging wedding dress once—but if you want long-lasting effects, you need to make long-term commitments.

So here's the deal. You follow the 14-day plan in order to drop a size for your own personal deadline—but once you've achieved your goal, you promise to read on to find out how you can take the lessons you've learned and make them fit into your lifestyle. Think of the 14 days as your launch pad to a healthier lifestyle. In section two, Habit Building, I'll show you how to incorporate the strategies and practices you've learned into your daily life, without feeling as if diet and exercise have taken over every waking minute. It's about taking things slowly and not trying to achieve everything all at once—it takes months for an action to become a habit, so you need to take it slowly and not try to do everything at once. Eventually, healthy living will become second nature. That doesn't mean there won't be times when you just can't avoid a blow-out, resist a fattening indulgence, or squeeze in an exercise session. We're all human, after all, and we have busy, unpredictable lives to lead. For this reason I've included section three, Damage Limitation, which shows you how to prevent the odd splurge from ruining all your good work.

Whatever your motivation is for losing weight fast, a forthcoming vacation, a family wedding, a party, or simply the thought of fitting back into your old jeans, it doesn't matter. If it provides the impetus for you to take action, then it has got to be a good thing. But sustaining that action for the rest of your life is the real key. It's not always easy, but you *can* do this, and there's no need to put your life on hold in order to achieve it. To help you toward your goals, you need information, inspiration, and encouragement. You'll find all three in this book—enabling you not only to lose weight in 14 days but also to keep it off for good.

Be active!

Joanna

DISCLAIMER: Please note that this diet and exercise plan is designed for people in good health and is not suitable for pregnant or nursing women. If there is any reason you think may prevent you following this diet and exercise plan safely, such as an existing health problem, something your doctor has told you, or feeling unwell, please consult your doctor before embarking on the program. The author(s) of this book cannot be held responsible for any health problems experienced as a result of following this diet or for any failure to lose weight. The plan is followed entirely at the participant's own risk.

SECTION ONE

So you're ready to drop a size,
we need to ...

GET A GRIP

THE 14-DAY GET A GRIP PLAN

ON YOUR MARKS

Right! We haven't got much time to spare if you're going to drop a size in 2 weeks flat, so read on to find out more about the plan and how to prepare, physically and psychologically, for the next 14 days.

WHY IS THE PLAN GOING TO WORK?

The 14-day plan combines diet and exercise. While weight loss can result from just dieting or just exercise, research has shown that a combination of both is the key to long-term results (it was also the ideal prescription for reducing blood pressure in a recent study). And it means you don't have to do either to the extreme—as both reduced energy intake and increased energy expenditure contribute to weight loss. Combining diet and exercise also helps to avoid the counterproductive changes to fat metabolism that can occur through dieting alone, according to a recent study published in the *American Journal of Clinical Nutrition*.

THE DIET PLAN

The eating plan is a carefully constructed low-calorie diet based on low glycemic index carbohydrates, to prevent the energy highs and lows that can lead to bingeing; dietary fiber, to help you feel satisfied; essential fatty acids for a healthy heart and efficient metabolic functioning; plenty of water-packed fruit, salad and vegetables to insure sufficient vitamin and mineral intake; and protein, essential for tissue repair, maintenance and growth.

The plan incorporates my Starch Curfew, a strategy that restricts carbohydrate intake after 5 p.m. to help you consume nutrients at the right time of day and maximize weight loss. It also has a high content of liquid-based foods, such as soups, stews and juices, because research has shown that these leave you feeling more satiated than a drier diet, even those that involve a high water intake. In one study, women who sipped a broth before they ate lunch consumed 100 fewer calories than those who did not—and felt less hungry later in the day.

The eating plan is easy to follow and clearly explained, with options for cooking at home as well as eating on the run, and while it is a low-calorie diet—providing approximately 1300 cals a day (1600 for men)—you can be assured that it's nutrient rich.

THE EXERCISE PLAN

Follow the 14-day eating plan and you'll soon be looking and feeling better. But for total health, vitality and successful weight loss, one crucial part of the jigsaw is still missing—exercise. Physical activity raises resting metabolism, increases calorie-hungry lean body mass, and improves your body's ability to burn fat as a fuel.

For convenience and simplicity, the aerobic exercise featured in the 14-day plan is simply walking. It's not only good for your figure but your health, too—recent research has shown that regular walking for as little as an hour a week is associated with lower incidence of heart disease in women. In the plan you will find that 10- to 30-minute bouts of walking are suggested at specific times during the day, but if you really can't fit them in, then stick to one daily walk. Some research shows that doing repeated bouts of exercise actually burns *more* calories than doing one prolonged session, due to the effect of exercise on metabolism, but the overall rule is to be as active as you can, as often as you can. There are daily step targets to aim for, to provide a guide to how much walking you need to do during the 14 days to get results. You'll need a pedometer—these are available for $10–$35 from good athletic equipment stores.

The daily walking is complemented by a targeted 10-minute home routine of abdominal and core stability exercises to tone up your abdominals and improve posture, all helping you to streamline your silhouette.

Alongside the walking and core exercises, try to find time to fit more "lifestyle" activity into each of the 14 days. These are activities that can be easily incorporated into your day and don't require you to get into your gym clothes and sneakers. Here are some everyday tasks that will help increase calorie expenditure.

Burn 100 calories without exercising by ...

Shopping for half an hour
Gardening for 20 minutes
Dancing for 20 minutes
Making the bed 5 days a week
Walking up stairs for 10 minutes
Cooking for 40 minutes
Cleaning for 25 minutes

ARE YOU READY TO DROP A DRESS SIZE?

Before you start, get a piece of paper and write down your answers to the following questions:

- Why do you want to drop a size? Try to think of at least three reasons.
- Do you have a particular deadline or event in mind? If so, write it down.

- Why do you think you have failed with previous weight loss attempts?
- What will be different this time?
- Are you willing to add daily activity to your life? Think of three ways you could add even just a little more physical activity to your daily routine.
- How do you think being slimmer, fitter, and healthier will affect your life?

Hopefully, the answers to the above questions will have helped focus your mind on the task in hand a little. Research shows that people who have an "intrinsic" or internal motivation to achieve something are more likely to persevere than those who are motivated by "extrinsic" rewards. For example, believing that you'll feel better about yourself if you drop a dress size is likely to help you stick with the plan more than having to lose weight for your best friend's wedding. It's important to be in the right frame of mind—positive, motivated, and confident—before you start and while on the *Get a Grip* plan. That's why you'll find a positive mantra and top tip for each day of your 14-day plan. It's also equally important to be practically and physically prepared. Make sure you have 14 days in which to commit yourself fully to this program—that means there should be no champagne-fueled parties or candle-lit dinners in your diary. Read through the next few pages and before you start make sure you have everything you need to make the plan a success.

IS MOTHER NATURE ON YOUR SIDE?

No matter how ready and willing you are to change your body, there are natural limitations that may influence your success. I call it the "Three M Theory"—your mother, your metabolism, and your motivation.

YOUR MOTHER

The way you were brought up can have a strong influence on your relationship with food later in life. Research from Pennsylvania State University showed that women who are faddy about foods tend to subconsciously pass on their finicky ways to their daughters. If your mother actively encouraged you not to eat certain foods or not to overeat, warning that it would make you fat, you probably label foods as "good" and "bad" without even realizing it. If you ate a lot of sweet and sugary things as you were growing up, and your diet didn't include a variety of tastes, it is likely that you now crave calorie-dense sweet foods rather than savory ones. Maybe your mother used to say "finish everything on your plate" and you still do. These attitudes have taken a long time to build into habits, and they will take a long time to diminish. This book will help you reevaluate your relationship with food, showing you how to draw up a sensible eating plan that will help you realize your weight and body fat goals, as well as providing a positive health message for your children.

YOUR METABOLISM

Research shows that from your mid-twenties onwards, metabolism begins to decline year on year. It's a sad fact that if you continue to consume the same number of calories without stepping up energy expenditure, gradual weight gain will result. In addition, there are specific times in life, for example during puberty, when fat cells are prone to get bigger and multiply. If we eat excessively during these times, it is likely that the body fat laid down in the fat cells will pose more of a problem to shift than the weight we gain at other times of our lives. This helps to explain why some friends appear to drop weight effortlessly while our own attempts require a lot more persistence. We are all designed to have fat cells, and they all have an ability to increase and decrease in size as we gain and lose weight. Appreciating this will allow you to approach this plan with a realistic picture of what you can achieve long term.

YOUR MOTIVATION

Consider this: what we weigh in seven years' time will not be determined by what we do in the next seven hours, seven days or seven weeks but by what we do consistently for the next seven years. So if your initial motivation to take those first steps is to get into a little black dress in 14 days' time—great! But once you've achieved that, use sections two and three to build on your success and make it last. Whatever your initial motivation to start the plan, try to find a way to translate it into a strategy that you can incorporate and build on to achieve your long-term weight and body fat goals. Establishing a strategy and action plan will be crucial, and the results that you'll see in 14 days will be the driving force to help you do so.

GET SET

This section is all about the practical stuff—what you need to buy, or have handy, how to take your current measurements (to help you gauge your results), and clear instructions on how to use the plan.

What you'll need:

- To take your current measurements you'll need a tape measure and a scale. If you don't have a scale, it's relatively easy to find one in a public place—try your local pool or drugstore.
- A pedometer to monitor the number of steps you take each day during the 14-day plan (you may wish to continue using it after the 14 days, too). These are available from most sports stores or sports product mail-order companies.
- A pair of good, supportive sneakers or walking shoes to wear on your daily ambles.
- For the abdominal and core stability exercises, you'll need some loose and comfortable clothing that doesn't restrict your movement. You won't work up a sweat, so don't

worry about changing into workout clothes unless you want to.

- One last thing you may consider purchasing is a juicer. These can be bought fairly cheaply from most department and electrical stores and give you access to a wider (and fresher) range of juices than relying on store-bought versions.

KITCHEN CABINET ESSENTIALS

This list serves as a general shopping list of non-perishable items that are used during the 14-day plan. There may be some other non-perishable items required for specific recipes, but the list below should cover you for most eventualities.

Oils, sauces and condiments

Olive oil
Oil cooking spray
Dijon mustard
Light soy sauce
Balsamic vinegar
White wine vinegar
Curry paste
Chicken or vegetable stock cubes
Red pesto
Arrabbiata sauce
Tabasco or any hot pepper/chili sauce
Tomato salsa
Mango chutney
Peanut butter
Honey

Herbs and spices

Mixed herbs
Root ginger
Fresh garlic bulbs
Ground cilantro
Ground cumin

Dried fruit and nuts

Sunflower seeds
Dried apricots
Unsalted almonds
Pine nuts

Cereals and cereal products

Oatmeal
Kelloggs All Bran
Post Fruit & Fibre
Crackers
Rice cakes

Beverages

Any herbal teas you enjoy
Soya milk

Cans

Chickpeas
Lentils
Chopped tomatoes
Anchovies
Tuna (in brine or spring water)
Butter beans
Flageolet beans
Corn
Baked beans (reduced salt and sugar)
Cannellini beans
Red kidney beans
Pink salmon

THE 14-DAY PLAN BASICS

Over the next few pages, you'll learn about the structure of the diet plan and how to use it. This is followed by each day of the plan clearly laid out with details of what to eat and when. You'll also find suggested "activity zones" in which to fit your walking or home exercises. You don't *have* to exercise at these times but it certainly helps to have some idea of when you're going to, rather than just leaving it to chance.

DAILY MUST-HAVES

Each day consists of breakfast, lunch and dinner; an energy-boosting "spruce juice"; a pre-dinner nutrient-packed "satisfying" soup, which you should aim to eat at least half an hour before you sit down for your main meal; and a snack.

The plan also includes the following "must-haves," which you should make sure you get each day:

- 1¼ cups of skimmed or semi-skimmed milk (if you are having milk in one of your meals, such as on breakfast cereal, it should come from this allowance). If you dislike, or are intolerant to milk, eat a 4oz pot of natural yogurt daily, or take a calcium supplement.
- 70oz (9 8-oz glasses) of water (spread evenly throughout the day—the plan suggests an appropriate time scale)
- a multi-vitamin tablet
- five servings of fruit and vegetables (see pages 32 and 113 to find out what the best options are)

The plan has been developed to provide a balanced intake of nutrients, vitamins and minerals. The breakfast for each day is listed in the plan, while you will find the lunch options on page 71 and the selection of Starch Curfew dinners on page 80. There are lunch and dinner options for vegetarians, fish and meat eaters—try to include as much variety as possible rather than sticking with the same thing every day. If you aren't vegetarian, try to consume three portions of oily fish each week.

SPRUCE JUICES

Your mid-morning spruce juice is specifically designed to boost energy levels, stabilize blood sugar until lunch, and pack a powerful nutrient punch for your body. The specific combination of vegetables and fruits has been selected to help cleanse your body and eliminate excess fluid and toxins from your body. Each juice is enough for two servings. You can either drink half in the morning and save the remaining half for your afternoon snack, or you can just make half of the recipe—whatever fits in with your day. If you don't have a juicer or blender, you can opt for store-bought juices or go to a juice bar and have one made up for you.

Celery, Beetroot, and Ginger Juice

You will need a juicer for this recipe.

½ bunch celery
¼ raw beetroot
1 cherry-sized piece fresh root ginger, peeled

Juice half the celery. Add the beetroot and ginger. Follow with the remaining celery.

Tomato, Parsley, and Pepper Juice

You can use a blender to make this juice.

14-oz can chopped tomatoes
large handful coarsely chopped parsley with stems
1 pepper, seeded and stem removed

Place the ingredients in a blender. Blend and enjoy.

Carrot, Apple, and Ginger Juice

You will need a juicer for this recipe.

4 carrots
2 apples
½-inch piece fresh root ginger, peeled

Combine the ingredients in a juicer.

Peach and Grape Nectar

Use a blender for this recipe.

1 large peach, pitted and coarsely chopped
2 good handfuls seedless green grapes

Blend and enjoy.

Summer Fruit Smoothie

Make this smoothie in a blender.

1 small banana, broken into chunks
1 peach, pitted and coarsely chopped
4 strawberries, washed and hulled, or use frozen strawberries
6 ice cubes
4¼-oz bottle raspberry drinking yogurt
¼ cup frozen low-fat vanilla yogurt

Blend the fruit in a blender with the ice cubes until smooth. Pour in the drinking yogurt and blend well. Pour into long glasses and add a scoop of vanilla yogurt to each glass.

Shop-bought alternatives:

- ⅔ cup unsweetened ready-packed carrot juice
- 1 small can V8
- ⅔ cup sugar- and additive-free fruit smoothie

SNACKS

When it comes to your mid-afternoon snack, we've left it up to you to choose from the list below, depending on how hungry you are and what you fancy. Each snack is approximately 100 calories.

- 1 cracker and 1 teaspoon peanut butter
- any piece of fruit (see the list on page 32 for suggestions if you're stuck in a Granny Smith rut!)
- 20 almonds
- 8 dried apricots
- 4oz pot low-fat yogurt and a small banana
- a palmful of sunflower and pumpkin seeds
- 2 rice cakes topped with cottage cheese
- half a small avocado filled with salsa
- 2 squares milk chocolate (Well, we are all human!)

SATISFYING SOUPS

Both these soups are filling and tasty and they'll provide your body with some of the essential nutrients it requires. Your daily soup should be taken pre-dinner, as this will fill you up and help stabilize blood sugar levels specifically when they may be starting to wane. This means you should feel more energized, less hungry, and less likely to overeat at your evening meal.

Full of Goodness (FOG) Soup

Makes 1 week's worth

Choose at least five of the vegetables listed below—the more the merrier! The initial preparation and cooking takes a little while but you then have a convenient soup that will last a week in the fridge—it freezes well too.

1 onion, coarsely chopped
1 zucchini, coarsely chopped
handful of green beans, cut into ½-inch lengths
1 carrot, diced
3 sticks celery, peeled with a potato peeler to remove the ridged strands and then coarsely chopped
1 leek, coarsely chopped
¼ cauliflower, cut into small bite-size pieces
4–5 green cabbage or spring green leaves, sliced into strips
1 small bunch broccoli, washed and cut into small bite-size pieces

1 parsnip, peeled and cut into bite-size pieces
14-oz can cannellini beans, drained and rinsed
handful of frozen peas
handful of snowpeas, diced
4–5 dried mushrooms, softened in 1¼ cups boiling water (the water can be added to the soup)
4 chicken or vegetable stock cubes
good handful of fresh chopped flat-leaf or curly parsley

Put all the vegetables, beans, and peas into a big stock pan together with the stock cubes and a gallon of cold water. Bring to a boil and then simmer on a very low heat, covered, for about 2 hours. Season well, halfway through cooking time.

Blend half of the soup in a blender or liquidizer and return it to the pot. Throw in the chopped parsley and serve.

Immune-boosting Soup

Makes enough for 1 week

This is a great detoxifying soup. It will cleanse your digestive system and is packed with antioxidants to boost your immune system.

2 teaspoons olive oil
2 carrots, chopped
2 onions, chopped
4 garlic cloves, crushed
2 red peppers, seeded and chopped
1 pinch ground allspice
1 tablespoon tomato purée
3 x 14-oz cans chopped tomatoes
1 chicken or vegetable stock cube dissolved
in 1¾ cups boiling water
2 cups freshly squeezed orange juice
4 tablespoons chopped fresh basil
salt and freshly ground black pepper

Heat the oil in a pan, add the carrot and onion and cook gently for 5 minutes. Add the garlic, red pepper, and ground allspice and cook for a further 3–4 minutes until the vegetables are tender. Add the tomato purée, chopped tomatoes, and stock and simmer for 10 minutes. Take off the heat and add the orange juice and chopped basil. Season well and serve.

A WORD ABOUT TEA, COFFEE, AND ALCOHOL

Finally, try to restrict coffee and tea intake to 2 cups a day. Herbal tea or green tea may be taken in any amount. In fact, one study from the University of Geneva found that green tea could boost metabolic rate by 4 percent. If you are a caffeine drinker, try to have your first cup of the day before you walk, and on an empty stomach, as studies have shown that caffeine enhances the utilization of fatty acids from the bloodstream, helping your body burn fat. Alcohol is not included in the 14-day plan. Not only is it calorie-rich and nutritionally poor, it also weakens your resolve and is likely to result in cheating, snacking, or going off the rails completely.

THE ABDOMINAL/CORE STABILITY EXERCISES

There are only four exercises in this home-based program—you could always do a lot more, but these exercises are designed to help you improve your posture and streamline your abdominals in minimum time. The idea is not to give you so many exercises that it stops you getting out and achieving your daily walking targets. For best results, I'd love you to do these six days a week—a day off gives your body a chance to rest and benefit from your efforts. If at all possible, do them in the morning. Research shows that people who exercise in the morning are more likely to stick with regular activity long term.

Do remember to warm up before you complete your exercises. In just 3–5 minutes you can mobilize your major joints and get rid of tension with brisk marching on the spot and running up and down stairs to increase your body temperature, shoulder rolls, some side bends, full-body stretches, a few squats, and knee lifts to your chest.

THE RIB–HIP CONNECTION

Master this technique to see great results in your abdominal/core stability exercises. When you lie on the floor, before you begin your abdominal work, make sure you have what is known as a "rib–hip connection". This will help you contract your abdominals before you lift and make sure your spine is in the correct anatomical position. Here is what to do: place your thumb on your bottom ribs and your fingers on the top of your hip bone and draw these two points together with a small contraction of your abdominal muscles. Your spine should be in a neutral position. This neutral position will vary from person to person dependent upon the shape of your spine. However, there should be a small space between the floor and your back. Keep the rib–hip connection so you maintain your neutral position. You are now ready to start your abdominal work.

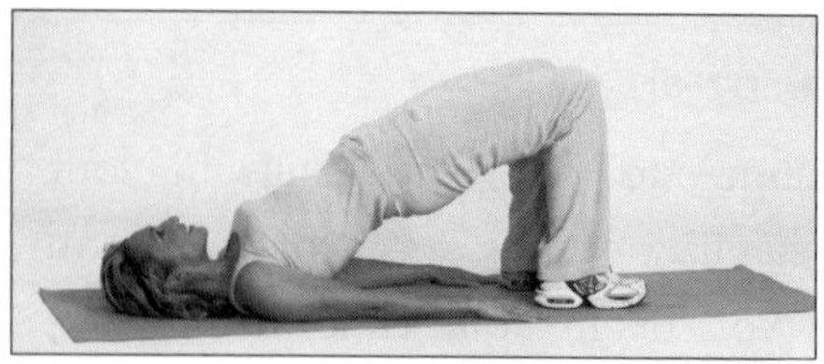

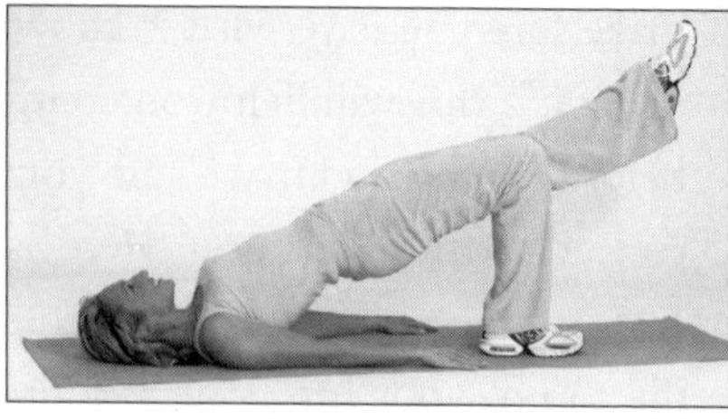

Exercise: The Bridge

What it does: Tightens your buttock muscles, flattens your abdominals, and strengthens your back.

Lie on your back, knees bent, feet flat on the floor, arms at your sides. Establish your rib–hip connection and use the hips, thigh, and trunk muscles to lift your pelvis off the floor until the body forms a diagonal line from your shoulders to your knees. Hold for 10 seconds. To make this exercise more challenging, extend one leg straight, hold for 4 counts, and lower to the ground. Now lift the other leg, hold for 4 counts, and lower to the ground. Now lower your whole body to the floor, still maintaining the rib–hip connection.

How many: Repeat 10 times

> **Joanna's top tip:** Visualizing pressing your knees away from your hips helps to stabilize your torso and tone your thighs.

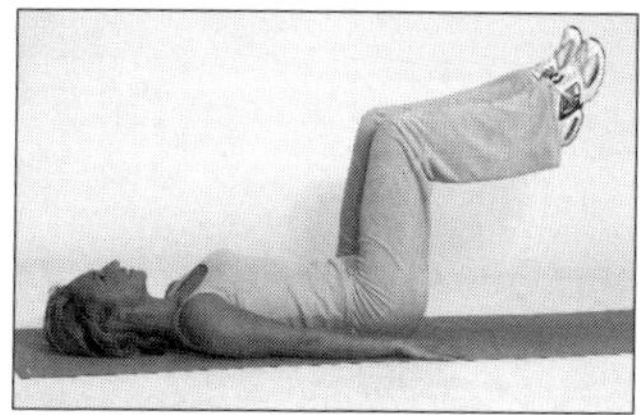

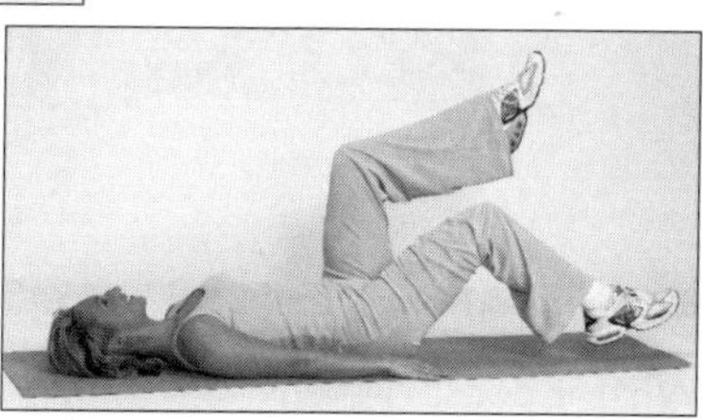

Exercise: Toe Touches

What it does: Flattens lower abdominal wall, especially the deep transverse muscle, which is crucial to getting that flatter tummy.

Lie on your back with knees over hips and lower legs parallel to the floor. Establish your rib–hip connection. Slowly lower one leg down to the floor, dropping your heel to the floor. Keep your spine in neutral as you lift your leg back over your chest. Repeat on the other side. The trick with this exercise is to go slowly and focus on technique. To make the exercise easier, bend your leg more and lower to the floor closer to your butt.

How many: Build up to 16 on each leg

> *Joanna's top tip:* This is a challenging exercise. Start out trying to do a few reps with really good technique. Remember the rib–hip connection.

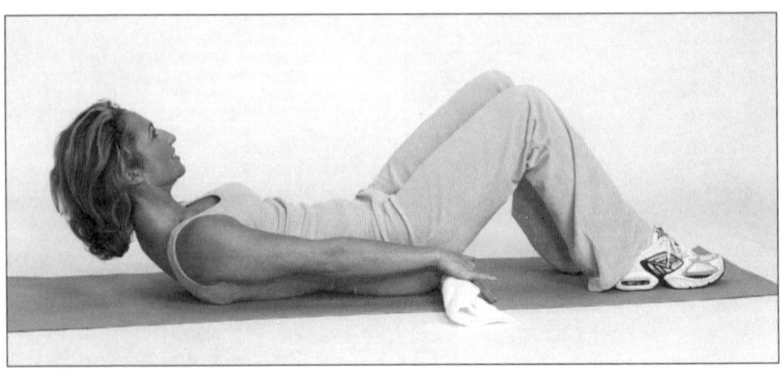

Exercise: Abdominal Curl Using a Towel

What it does: Tightens upper abdominals, especially around rib and upper waist area.

Lie on the floor, knees bent. Place a rolled towel between your butt and your feet, slightly in front of your extended fingers. Slide your feet away from your butt until you feel your toes start to come off the floor. Slowly curl up from your breastbone and lift your fingers over the top of the towel to touch the floor on the other side. The emphasis should be on tucking your ribs under rather than lifting up.

How many: 16–20 reps

> **Joanna's top tip:** This is especially good post-pregnancy, when the rib cage has often extended due to the growing baby. Imagine you are wearing a tight corset to help you draw down through your rib cage with each lift, but do remember to breathe.

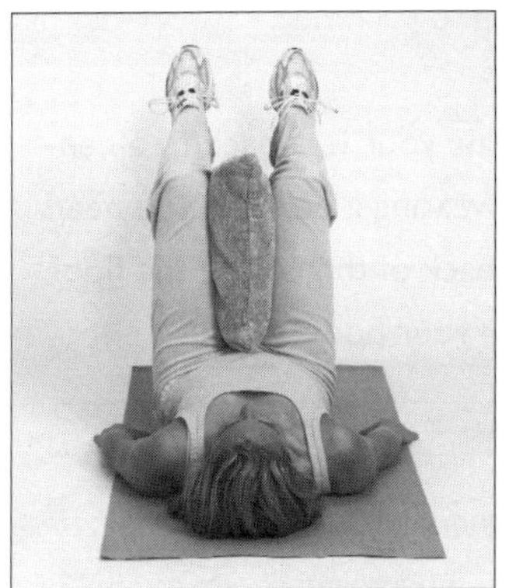
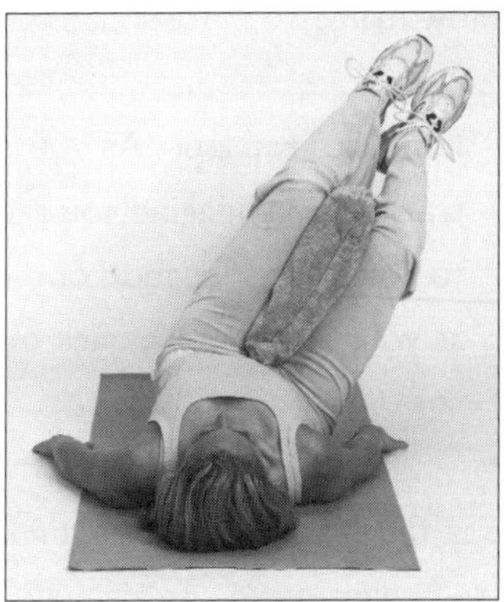

Exercise: Abdominal Pillow Rolls

What it does: Develops trunk stability and tones waist muscles.

Lie on the floor, knees bent and feet flat. Place a pillow or small cushion between your knees. Lightly squeeze the pillow between your knees as you lower your knees to one side. As you draw your knees back to a central position, focus on contracting your abdominals down to the floor and tightening your waist. To make the exercise more challenging, start with your legs lifted off the floor with your knees over your chest. Slowly lower your knees to one side but do not drop them to the floor, keep the rib–hip connection as you draw your abdominals back in, and focus on tightening around your waist muscles as you come back to a flat position.

How many: 16 in total, alternating to each side

> *Joanna's top tip:* **As you draw your legs back to a central position imagine you are wearing a belt and you need to flatten each section of the back of the belt to the floor as your knees move back over your body.**

See the Bonus Info Panels throughout the 14-day plan for troubleshooting tips on walking and the abdominal exercises.

GO!

Measure and weigh yourself at the start of day 1, in the morning *before* you eat or drink anything. Make a note of your measurements on the table below. See the guidelines on the following page for how to take your measurements precisely.

For Women	**For Men**
weight	weight
body fat (if known)	body fat (if known)
chest	chest
waist	waist: bellybutton contracted
navel	waist: bellybutton relaxed
hips	hips
thighs	thighs

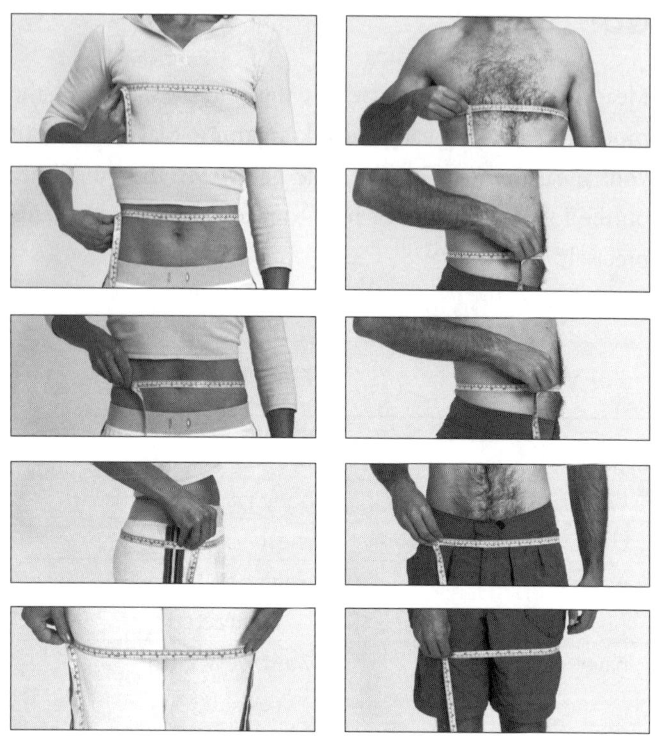

HOW TO MEASURE

Chest—measure with the tape flat across the nipple line

Waist—measure around the narrowest part of your midriff (for men, pull your tummy in for the first reading and let it go for the second)

Navel—measure around the midriff directly over the bellybutton

Hips—measure across the top of the buttock cheeks

Thighs—standing with feet together, measure 20cm up from the top of your kneecap and take a circumference measurement of your thighs.

DAY 1

Today's mantra: *This is about me taking the first steps to a healthier life.*

Today's step target: 7000

Tip/testimony from volunteer: *For years I tried different dieters' classes and quick-fix programs but what I really needed was education. By developing an understanding of the foods I should be avoiding and those I should be increasing, and learning to fit structured exercise around my family, I feel like I can achieve my goal at last.* **Vickie, 29**

On rising	1 glass of water plus cup of coffee, green tea or tea, or hot water and lemon
Suggested activity zone	15-minute walk (step target 1800) plus abdominal and core stability exercises (see page 22)
Breakfast	2 glasses of water breakfast cereal: ½ cup bran cereal or ⅓ cup bran cereal and dried fruit with ⅔ cup semi-skimmed milk and ½ cup raspberries 1 glass apple juice
Mid-morning spruce juice	choose a juice from those listed on page 14
Suggested activity zone	15-minute walk (step target 1800)
Lunch	1 glass of water a lunch from the options suggested on pages 71–9

Mid-afternoon snack	2 glasses of water a snack from the options listed on page 17
Suggested activity zone	20-minute walk (step target 2400)
Satisfying soup	choose either the FOG or Immune-boosting Soup—make enough to last at least a few days (see page 20)
Dinner	2 glasses of water a Starch Curfew meal from the selection on pages 80–97
Suggested activity zone	10-minute walk (step target 1000)
Bedtime drink	chamomile tea, hot milk or soya milk, or hot water and lemon

TOP FRUIT

Not all fruit are created equal when it comes to cutting calories and boosting nutrients. The list below features the top water-dense fruits and what constitutes a serving of each.

Fruit	1 serving
Kiwi	2 fruits
Strawberries	large cup
Orange	1 large
Melon (any variety)	cereal bowl
Grapefruit	large cup
Raspberries	large cup
Pears	1 large
Grapes	large cup
Blueberries	large cup

DAY 2

Today's mantra: *Every small thing I do matters.*

Today's step target: 8000

Tip/testimony from volunteer: *It was hard to fit in all the walks with my day-to-day lifestyle but I adapted the activity zones to suit my own life and made sure I fitted in as much activity as possible. I definitely feel fitter.* **Melanie, 39**

On rising	1 glass of water plus cup of coffee, green tea or tea, or hot water and lemon
Suggested activity zone	15-minute walk (step target 1800) plus abdominal and core stability exercises (see page 22)
Breakfast	2 glasses of water 3 rye crispbread with 1 mashed banana and 2T peanut butter cup of tea or coffee
Mid-morning spruce juice	choose a juice from those listed on page 14
Suggested activity zone	15-minute walk (step target 1800)
Lunch	1 glass of water a lunch from the options suggested on pages 71–9
Mid-afternoon snack	2 glasses of water snack a snack from the options listed on page 17

Suggested activity zone	20-minute walk (step target 2500)
Satisfying soup	1 bowl of FOG or Immune-boosting Soup
Dinner	2 glasses of water a Starch Curfew meal from the selection on pages 80–97
Suggested activity zone	15-minute walk (step target 1800–1900)
Bedtime drink	chamomile tea, hot milk or soya milk, or hot water and lemon

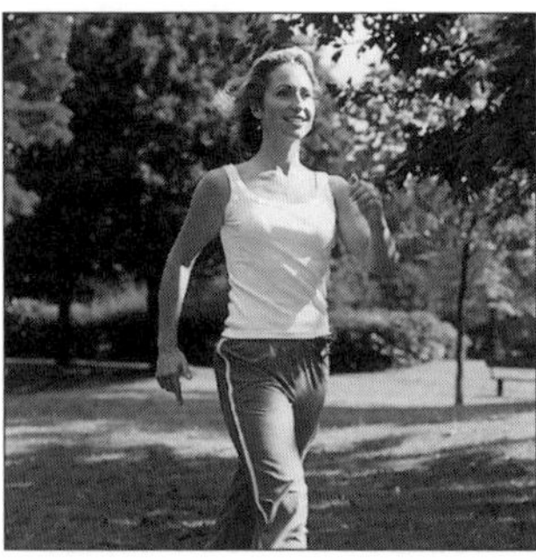

TIPS ON WALKING TECHNIQUE

Start slowly to give your body a chance to adapt to the demands of walking. Once you're in full swing, bear in mind the following tips:

- Land on your heel and roll through to push off with the forefoot
- Don't overstride—shorter, quicker strides are more natural
- Keep your abdominals gently contracted, your chest lifted and shoulders relaxed as you walk
- Swing your arms with approximately a right angle at the elbow joint, swinging them faster to speed up your walking pace.

DAY 3

Today's mantra: I feel energized

Today's step target: 9000

Tip/testimony from volunteer: *Read the whole day's eating plan first thing so you have time to stock up and/or make contingency plans for anything you don't like to eat or won't have time to cook.* **Sam, 33**

On rising	1 glass of water plus cup of coffee, green tea or tea, or hot water and lemon
Suggested activity zone	15-minute walk (step target 1800) plus abdominal and core stability exercises (see page 22)
Breakfast	2 glasses of water fruit and yoghurt: chop up 1 apple, 1 peach, 1 pear and 1 plum (or substitute ⅓ cup of red grapes for any of these), add a 4oz pot of natural yogurt and sprinkle with a tablespoon of sunflower seeds
Mid-morning spruce juice	choose a juice from those listed on page 14
Suggested activity zone	15-minute walk (step target 1800–2000)
Lunch	1 glass of water a lunch from the options suggested on pages 71–9
Mid-afternoon snack	2 glasses of water a snack from the options listed on page 17

Suggested activity zone	30-minute walk (step target 3600)
Satisfying soup	1 bowl of FOG or Immune-boosting soup
Dinner	2 glasses of water a Starch Curfew meal from the selection on pages 80–97
Suggested activity zone	15-minute walk (step target 1800)
Bedtime drink	chamomile tea, hot milk or soya milk, or hot water and lemon

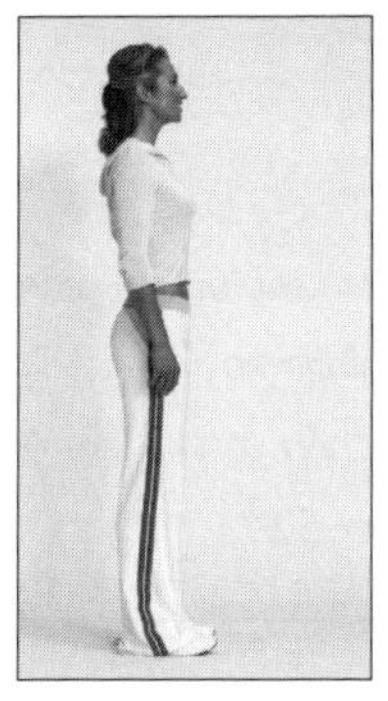

PERFECT POSTURE

The way we stand says a lot about us. It can portray our emotions as well as the general health of our bodies. Lifestyles today erode our natural ability for good posture—driving for hours or spending all day at a desk can all affect our posture. Long term, these misalignments can have a big impact on the health of our spines. Safeguarding your spine and posture does not require a large investment in terms of time.

To perfect your posture, stand with your feet hip-distance apart with your weight evenly distributed. Soften your knees as you pull up through your legs. Keep the hips square and level. Lengthen through the spine and contract the abdominals, sucking the belly button into the back of the spine as you extend tall. Drop the rib cage, pulling the lower ribs towards the pubic bone. The shoulders should be down and relaxed, so the neck is as long as possible. Breathe smoothly.

DAY 4

Today's mantra: I feel strong and focused.

Today's step target: 10,000

Tip/testimony from volunteer: *When you first set out to lose weight, keep as busy as possible with other things so you don't keep thinking about it—and keep out of the kitchen so you aren't tempted to open the fridge all the time!* **Robyn, 52**

On rising	1 glass of water plus cup of coffee, green tea or tea, or hot water and lemon
Suggested activity zone	15-minute walk (step target 1800–2000) plus abdominal and core stability exercises (see page 22)
Breakfast	2 glasses of water 1 grapefruit followed by 1 slice of stoneground, wholewheat bread with a scrape of butter and yeast extract
Mid-morning spruce juice	choose a juice from those listed on page 14
Suggested activity zone	20-minute walk (step target 2400)
Lunch	1 glass of water a lunch from the options suggested on pages 71–9
Mid-afternoon snack	2 glasses of water a snack from the options listed on page 17

Suggested activity zone	30-minute walk (step target 3600)
Satisfying soup	1 bowl of FOG or Immune-boosting soup
Dinner	2 glasses of water a Starch Curfew meal from the selection on pages 80–97
Suggested activity zone	15–20-minute walk (step target 2200)
Bedtime drink	chamomile tea, hot milk or soya milk, or hot water and lemon

ABDOMINAL EXERCISE TROUBLESHOOTING

Problem: lower tummy muscles "popping out"

Sometimes as we lift, the lower abdominal muscles can "pop" out. This can create less stability in the lower back as well as not helping to flatten the abdominal wall. **Here are a couple of solutions to help train the abdominal wall to flatten.**

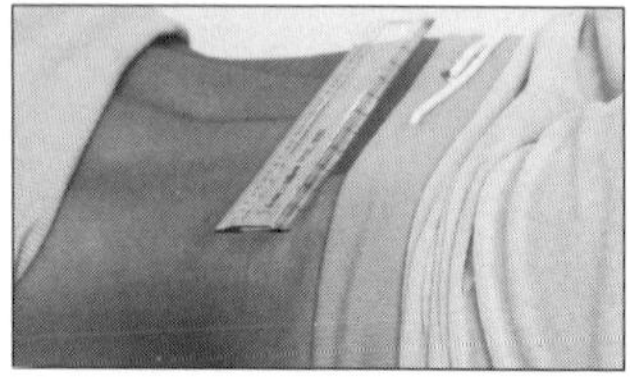

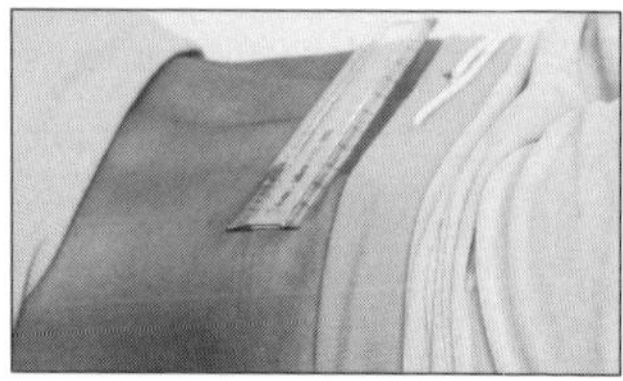

1. Check you have rib–hip connection (see page 23) then place a ruler across your lower abdominal muscles. As you lift, try to keep the ruler in place by focusing on drawing down through the lower abdominal wall—the ruler just gives you a reminder of how to do this.

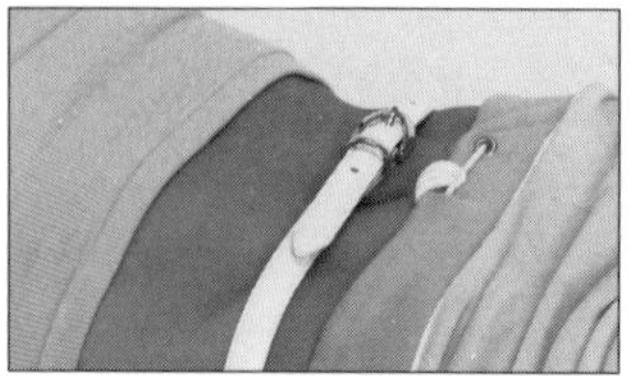

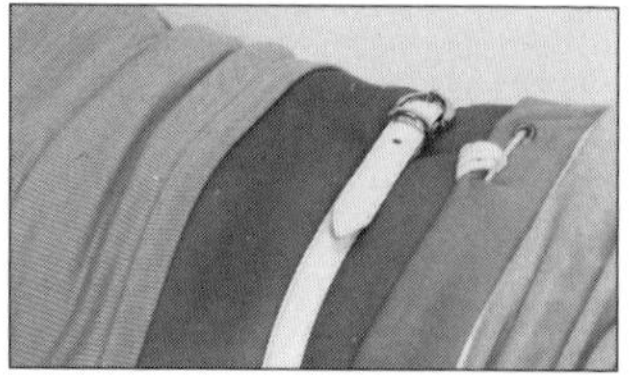

2. Wear a belt for your abdominal exercises. Buckle it so you have a little movement between your abdominals and the belt. As you lift, focus on keeping your abdominals away from the belt buckle and not pressing against it.

DAY 5

Today's mantra: *My body feels tall and poised.*

Today's step target: 10,000

Tip/testimony from volunteer: *When I first started the plan I had to completely re-think my eating habits. Towards the end of the first week I was getting to grips with it—I'd lost 3lb and my energy levels were increasing.* **Elaine, 33**

On rising	1 glass of water plus cup of coffee, green tea or tea, or hot water and lemon
Suggested activity zone	15-minute walk (step target 1800) plus abdominal and core stability exercises (see page 22)
Breakfast	2 glasses of water porridge: ⅔ cup oatmeal cooked with ⅔ cup of semi-skimmed milk and garnished with 4 chopped dried apricots cup of tea or coffee
Mid-morning spruce juice	choose a juice from those listed on page 14
Suggested activity zone	20-minute walk (step target 2400)
Lunch	1 glass of water a lunch from the options suggested on pages 71–9
Mid-afternoon snack	2 glasses of water a snack from the options listed on page 17

Suggested activity zone	30-minute walk (step target 3600)
Satisfying soup	1 bowl of FOG or Immune-boosting soup
Dinner	2 glasses of water a Starch Curfew meal from the selection on pages 80–97
Suggested activity zone	15–20-minute walk (step target 2200)
Bedtime drink	chamomile tea, hot milk or soya milk, or hot water and lemon

STRETCHES FOR WALKING

It's important to stretch out your muscles after walking, to reduce stiffness, maintain flexibility and aid recovery. Here are some of the key stretches you may find helpful.

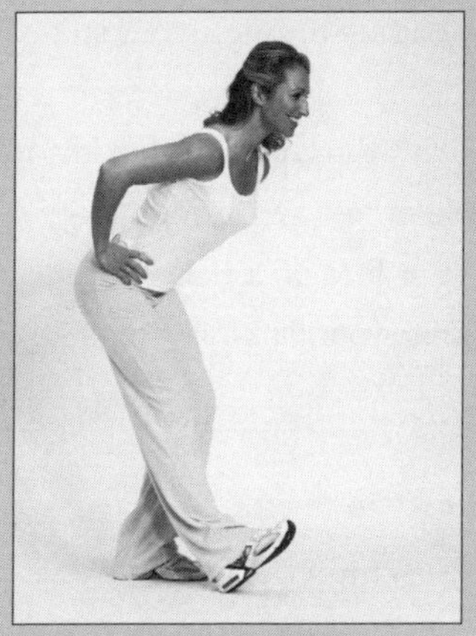

Standing Hamstring Stretch

Stand with good posture. Extend one leg out in front of you with the heel on the floor. Bend the back knee and flex forward from the hips. Make sure you contract your abdominals as you extend forward. Lift up out of the hips and check they are level. Imagine you need to balance two glasses of water on each side of your lower back to help you.

Joanna's top tip: To progress the stretch, lift your leg and rest it on a bench or low step or chair. Lift your tailbone up behind you to feel a greater stretch.

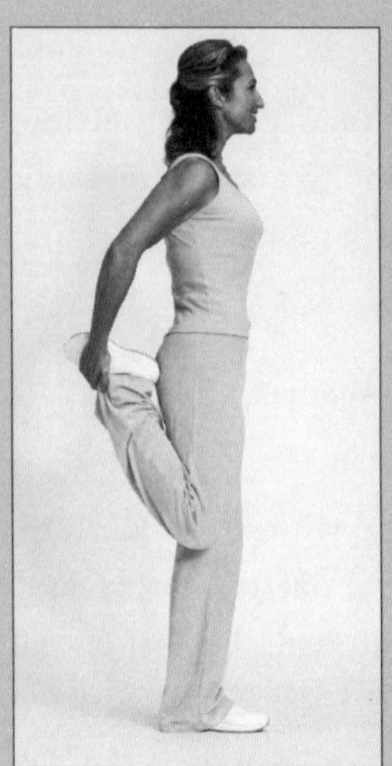

Standing Quad Stretch

Stand with good posture. Lift one leg, bending at the knee, and hold the laces of your shoe in your hand. Keep the knees together. Gently press your hips forward as you extend up through your spine.

Joanna's top tip: If you are less flexible or feel pain in your knee, rest your foot on a chair instead and press your hips forward.

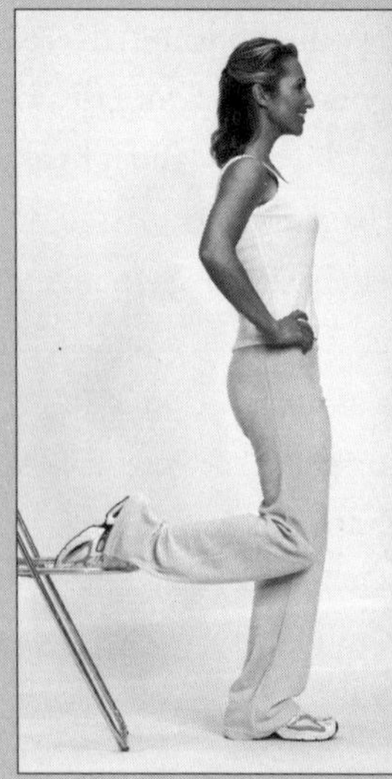

Standing Hip Flexor Stretch

Start in a lunge position. Make sure your front knee is over your ankle and your kneecap is in line with your second toe. Extend the back leg, and push the pelvis forward, using a chair for support or placing both hands on your front leg.

Joanna's top tip: Keep the body upright rather than leaning forward. Drawing up through your pelvic floor muscle will help with your balance.

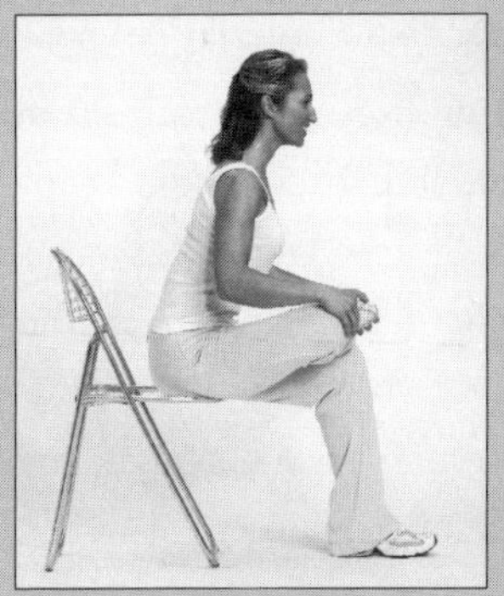

Seated Buttock Stretch

Sit on the edge of a chair with good posture. Place your arms on the back of the chair, fingers pointing back. Cross one ankle and rest the leg on the other knee. To progress this stretch, place your hands on the side of the chair. Support your body weight and lift yourself off the chair, slowly lowering yourself toward the floor. You should feel a deep stretch on the buttock of the crossed leg.

Joanna's top tip: Make sure you extend through your spine as you sit. If you suffer from knee pain, try the lying buttock stretch instead.

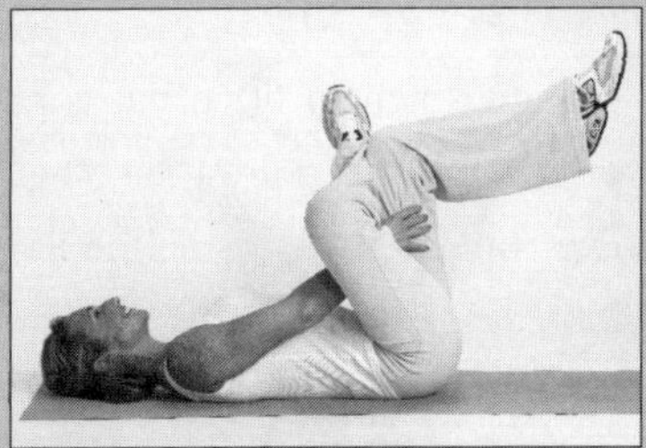

Lying Buttock and Hip Stretch

Lie on your back with neutral posture, abdominals contracted and knees bent. Cross one ankle over and rest it on your knee. You may feel a stretch in this position. To increase the stretch, draw one knee into the chest, holding behind the thigh. If you are very flexible you may need to take the supporting leg slightly closer to the chest to feel the stretch.

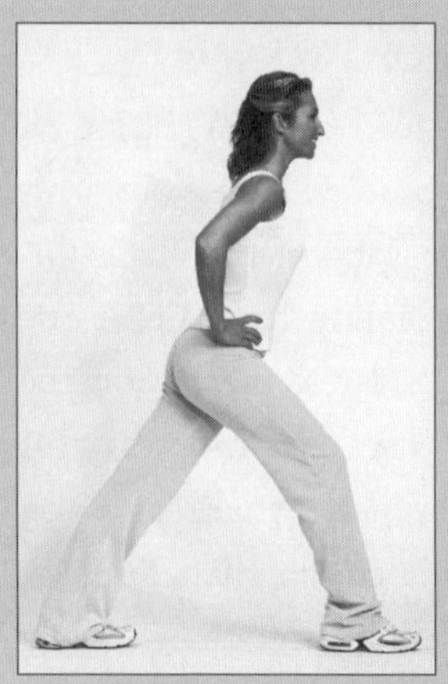

Standing Calf Stretch

Stand with good posture. Take a large step backwards, keeping both feet facing forwards and the front knee over the ankle. If you draw an imaginary line down through the middle of the kneecap it would be in line with the second toe. Press the back heel down to the floor. Make sure the body is in line from the top of your head to your back foot. Use a wall for support if you need to.

Joanna's top tip: To stretch more into the lower calf, bring the back leg in a little and bend the back leg at the knee.

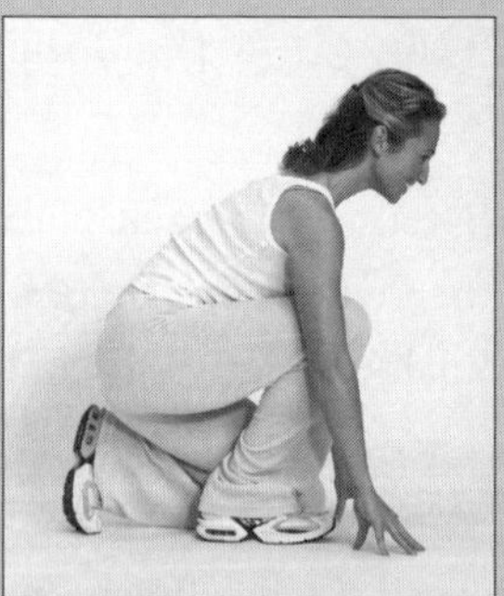

Achilles Stretch

Crouch down to place one foot on the ground and rest the other knee on the floor beside the flat foot. Keep the foot flat on the floor and lean forward over your knee until you feel a stretch on the Achilles of that foot.

Joanna's top tip: Press the front knee forward and diagonally toward the floor to feel a more effective Achilles stretch. This is a good stretch to do if you are a lover of high heels!

DAY 6

Today's mantra: I can do this!

Today's step target: 10,000

Tip/testimony from volunteer: *My mood was excellent while I was following the plan, which surprised me because I've always felt irritable when I've tried to lose weight before. I felt good because I was actually doing something about my weight and my health.* **Joan, 63**

On rising	1 glass of water plus cup of coffee, green tea or tea, or hot water and lemon
Suggested activity zone	15-minute walk (step target 1800) plus abdominal and core stability exercises (see page 22)
Breakfast	2 glasses of water baked beans on toast: warm a small can (⅔ cup) of baked beans and serve on 2 small slices of rye bread
Mid-morning spruce juice	choose a juice from those listed on page 14
Suggested activity zone	20-minute walk (step target 2400)
Lunch	1 glass of water a lunch from the options suggested on pages 71–9
Mid-afternoon snack	2 glasses of water a snack from the options listed on page 17

Suggested activity zone 30-minute walk (step target 3600)

Satisfying soup 1 bowl of FOG or Immune-boosting soup

Dinner 2 glasses of water
a Starch Curfew meal from the selection on pages 80–97

Suggested activity zone 15–20-minute walk (step target 2200)

Bedtime drink chamomile tea, hot milk or soya milk, or hot water and lemon

UNLIMITED VEGETABLES AND SALADS

All the lunches and dinners can be accompanied by as much as you want of the following vegetables or salad. Do not, however, add extra calories by stir-frying or coating them with dressing!

Choose from the following list:

asparagus
cabbage
spring greens
kale
spinach
mushrooms
fennel
tomatoes
squash
cucumber
celery
onions
red, yellow, and green peppers
leeks
lettuce and all other salad greens
zucchini

DAY 7

Today's mantra: Taking action is making me feel better about myself.

Today's step target: 7000

Tip/testimony from volunteer: *Don't be despondent if the weight doesn't come off right away. I found the real difference came during the last few days of the plan.* **Melanie, 30**

On rising	1 glass of water plus cup of coffee, green tea or tea, or hot water and lemon
Suggested activity zone	30-minute walk (step target 3500)
Breakfast	2 glasses of water breakfast grill: broil 3 tomatoes and a handful of mushrooms (sprayed with oil) and serve with 1 poached egg and a slice of wholewheat toast
Mid-morning spruce juice	choose a juice from those listed on page 14
Suggested activity zone	rest
Lunch	1 glass of water a lunch from the options suggested on pages 71–9
Mid-afternoon snack	2 glasses of water a snack from the options listed on page 19

Suggested activity zone	rest
Satisfying soup	1 bowl of FOG or Immune-boosting soup
Dinner	2 glasses of water a Starch Curfew meal from the selection on pages 80–97
Suggested activity zone	30-minute walk (step target 3500)
Bedtime drink	chamomile tea, hot milk or soya milk, or hot water and lemon

THE IMPORTANCE OF REST

Did you notice that today's walking schedule is a bit easier? Everyone needs time to recover and adapt to new demands and that's why the plan incorporates this easier day. This is the perfect time to reward yourself for the hard work you've done so far with a relaxing hot bath, a massage or simply putting your feet up with a good book. You'll also feel refreshed and motivated to get back to business tomorrow.

DAY 8

Today's mantra: *Today is a new day and I feel great.*
Today's step target: 10,000
Tip/testimony from volunteer: *At first, my skin got worse and I caught a cold but my pimples soon vanished and I didn't have any stomach problems, which I normally have on a regular basis. By the end of the 14 days my stomach was much flatter and I had lost inches.* **Natasha, 28**

On rising	1 glass of water plus cup of coffee, green tea or tea, or hot water and lemon
Suggested activity zone	15-minute walk (step target 1800) plus abdominal and core stability exercises (see page 22)
Breakfast	2 glasses of water porridge: ⅔ cup oatmeal cooked with ⅔ cup semi-skimmed milk and garnished with 4 chopped dried apricots cup of tea or coffee
Mid-morning spruce juice	choose a juice from those listed on page 14
Suggested activity zone	20-minute walk (step target 2400)
Lunch	1 glass of water a lunch from the options suggested on pages 71–9
Mid-afternoon snack	2 glasses of water a snack from the options listed on page 19

Suggested activity zone	30-minute walk (step target 3600)
Satisfying soup	1 bowl of FOG or Immune-boosting soup
Dinner	2 glasses of water a Starch Curfew meal from the selection on pages 80–97
Suggested activity zone	15–20-minute walk (step target 2200)
Bedtime drink	chamomile tea, hot milk or soya milk, or hot water and lemon

NOT BOTHERING WITH THE BEDTIME DRINK?

You may find the bedtime drink helps you sleep better and wake up refreshed. Warm fluids are more soothing than cold drinks at this time, when you want your body to relax. Milky drinks, including soya-based ones, are a good source of the amino acid tryptophan, consumption of which can boost brain serotonin levels, leaving you feeling relaxed and sleepy. Chamomile is a soothing herb, which can aid relaxation and help banish insomnia. If nothing else, your bedtime drink will add to your daily hydration.

DAY 9

Today's mantra: *I am feeling stronger and fitter.*
Today's step target: 10,000
Tip/testimony from volunteer: *Even on days when I didn't have time to fit in all the activity zones, I tried to do something—even 10 minutes is better than nothing at all.* **Sharon, 26**

On rising	1 glass of water plus cup of coffee, green tea or tea, or hot water and lemon
Suggested activity zone	15-minute walk (step target 1800) plus abdominal and core stability exercises (see page 22)
Breakfast	2 glasses of water fruit and yogurt: chop up 1 apple, 1 peach, 1 pear and 1 plum (or substitute ⅔ cup of red grapes for any of these), add a 4oz pot of natural yogurt and sprinkle with a tablespoon of sunflower seeds
Mid-morning spruce juice	choose a juice from those listed on page 14
Suggested activity zone	20-minute walk (step target 2400)
Lunch	1 glass of water a lunch from the options suggested on pages 71–9
Mid-afternoon snack	2 glasses of water a snack from the options listed on page 19

Suggested activity zone	30-minute walk (step target 3600)
Satisfying soup	1 bowl of FOG or Immune-boosting soup
Dinner	2 glasses of water a Starch Curfew meal from the selection on pages 80–97
Suggested activity zone	15–20-minute walk (step target 2200)
Bedtime drink	chamomile tea, hot milk or soya milk, or hot water and lemon

ABDOMINAL WORK TROUBLESHOOTING

Problem: Neck Pain

Many people put off doing abdominal exercises as they complain of feeling neck pain. This generally relates to the fact that the abdominals are weak and the neck muscles are helping to lift the body up. **Here are two quick and simple solutions to relieve discomfort and safeguard your neck as you build up strength, tone and flatten your abdominals.**

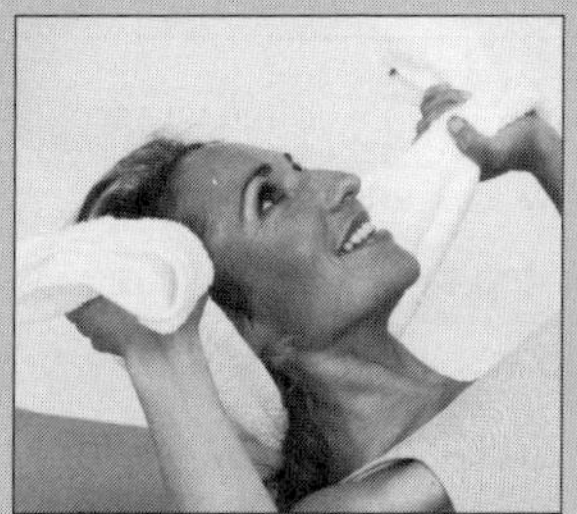

1. Take a towel and place behind the head. Hold both ends taut so it supports the neck. Keep the towel taut as you curl up and down.

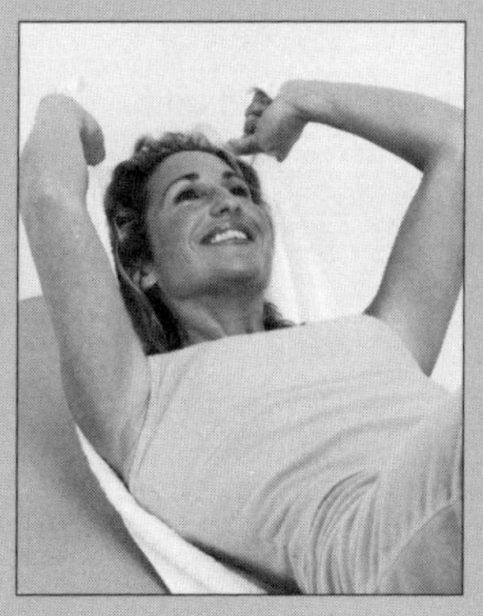

2. Place a towel open on the floor and lie on it so the back of your ribs secures the bottom of the towel to the floor. Reach your arms above your head, hold onto the ends of the towel with your hands and pull it taut as you complete your curls.

DAY 10

Today's mantra: *I feel really proud of my actions.*

Today's step target: 10,000

Tip/testimony from volunteer: *Before I started the plan, I would often feel hungry between meals and have some chips or candy. I've found that drinking 2½ quarts of water a day suppresses the need to eat when I'm not genuinely hungry. I was amazed by what this simple action did for my hunger and energy!* **Alec, 33**

On rising	1 glass of water plus cup of coffee, green tea or tea, or hot water and lemon
Suggested activity zone	15-minute walk (step target 1800) plus abdominal and core stability exercises (see page 22)
Breakfast	2 glasses of water 1 grapefruit followed by a slice of stoneground wholewheat bread with a scrape of butter and yeast extract
Mid-morning spruce juice	choose a juice from those listed on page 14
Suggested activity zone	20-minute walk (step target 2400)
Lunch	1 glass of water a lunch from the options suggested on pages 71–9
Mid-afternoon snack	2 glasses of water a snack from the options listed on page 19

Suggested activity zone	30-minute walk (step target 3600)
Satisfying soup	1 bowl of FOG or Immune-boosting soup
Dinner	2 glasses of water a Starch Curfew meal from the selection on pages 80–97
Suggested activity zone	15–20-minute walk (step target 2200)
Bedtime drink	chamomile tea, hot milk or soya milk, or hot water and lemon

SORE SHINS?

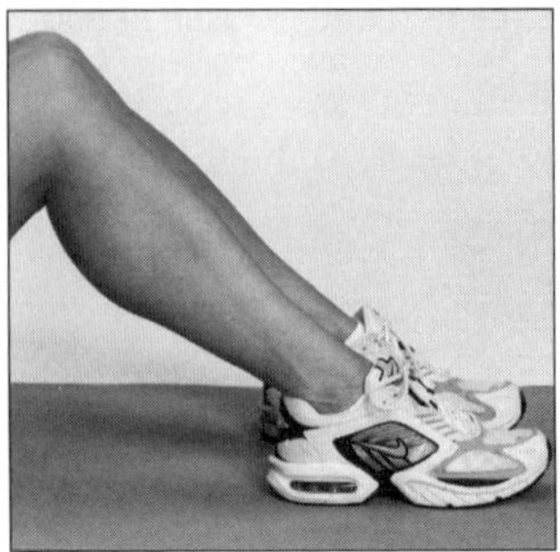

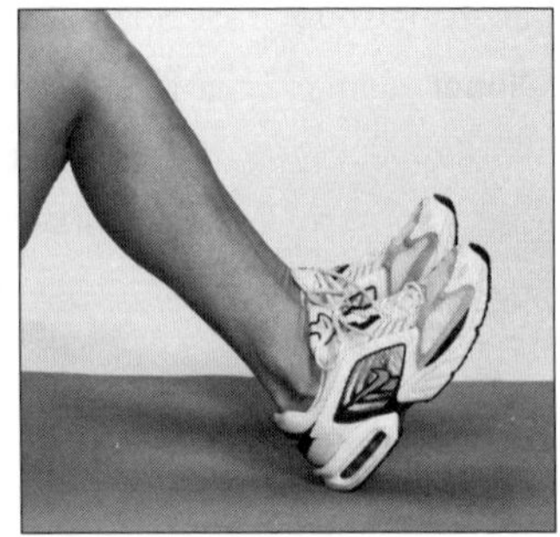

If you're not accustomed to walking, you may find that the area along the front of your shins is sore or tender, particularly if you've been walking mainly on hard surfaces like concrete. This soreness is usually a result of inflammation of the anterior tibialis muscles, which lie along the front of the shin. These muscles are often weak and are prone to inflammation when we increase their usage.

To combat this problem, try this shin-strengthening exercise.

Lie on your back, knees bent, feet flat on the floor. Lift your toes off the floor, drawing them into your shins. The heels stay on the floor. Hold for 10 seconds and release. To make this harder you can attach a dynaband over the top of the foot and secure against a post as you lift your foot—you will then have the extra resistance of the band to work against.

DAY 11

Today's mantra: I feel in control.

Today's step target: 10,000

Tip/testimony from volunteer: *The hardest recommendation to follow for me was to exercise. I now exercise every day for at least 30 minutes, including a speed walk/jog first thing in the morning. That alone means I start the day with a strong sense of positive achievement.* **Vanessa, 55**

On rising	1 glass of water plus cup of coffee, green tea or tea, or hot water and lemon
Suggested activity zone	15-minute walk (step target 1800) plus abdominal and core stability exercises (see page 22)
Breakfast	2 glasses of water apricot and banana smoothie: soften 6 dried apricots in boiling water, then place a ripe banana, a 4oz pot of natural yogurt, a spoonful of honey and ⅔ cup semi-skimmed milk into a blender, add the softened apricots and blend until smooth
Mid-morning spruce juice	choose a juice from those listed on page 14
Suggested activity zone	20-minute walk (step target 2400)
Lunch	1 glass of water a lunch from the options suggested on pages 71–9

Mid-afternoon snack	2 glasses of water a snack from the options listed on page 19
Suggested activity zone	30-minute walk (step target 3600)
Satisfying soup	1 bowl of FOG or Immune-boosting soup
Dinner	2 glasses of water a Starch Curfew meal from the selection on pages 80–97
Suggested activity zone	15–20-minute walk (step target 2200)
Bedtime drink	chamomile tea, hot milk or soya milk, or hot water and lemon

EAT TO GET SLIM

If you've followed the plan correctly it's likely that you haven't felt hungry. You may even have felt tempted to skip your spruce juice or miss out an afternoon snack. After all, the more calories you can cut, the better, right? Wrong! The very process of digestion actually increases your metabolism and contributes significantly—roughly 5 percent—to your daily energy expenditure. So skipping meals and snacks denies your body the chance to rev up its metabolism in order to digest them. If you feel over-full and really don't want to eat as much as is suggested, try reducing the amounts at *all* meals rather than cutting out specific ones altogether.

DAY 12

Today's mantra: *I feel like a new person!*
Today's step target: 10,000
Tip/testimony from volunteer: *Don't get disheartened if, from time to time, you fail to stick with the plan. A realistic and flexible approach is just as important as being disciplined.* **Tom, 29**

On rising	1 glass of water plus cup of coffee, green tea or tea, or hot water and lemon
Suggested activity zone	15-minute walk (step target 1800) plus abdominal and core stability exercises (see page 22)
Breakfast	2 glasses of water 3 rye crispbread with 1 mashed banana and 2 tablespoons peanut butter cup of tea or coffee
Mid-morning spruce juice	choose a juice from those listed on page 14
Suggested activity zone	20-minute walk (step target 2400)
Lunch	1 glass of water a lunch from the options suggested on pages 71–9
Mid-afternoon snack	2 glasses of water a snack from the options listed on page 19
Suggested activity zone	30-minute walk (step target 3600)

Satisfying soup	1 bowl of FOG or Immune-boosting soup
Dinner	2 glasses of water a Starch Curfew meal from the selection on pages 80–97
Suggested activity zone	15–20-minute walk (step target 2200)
Bedtime drink	chamomile tea, hot milk or soya milk, or hot water and lemon

EVERY STEP COUNTS

Walking is about the best exercise we can do. It is the simplest, least expensive and most effective exercise for the vast majority of individuals. The health benefits of walking have been known for a long time, but now research has quantified the number of walking steps we should be taking each day to achieve specific activity goals. It has been shown that 4000 steps a day is the minimum we should all be taking to have a positive impact on our health, whereas 7000 steps a day can positively improve our fitness levels and 10,000 steps a day can contribute to weight loss. Hopefully, you're beginning to see opportunities for quick walks throughout the day, so that you can break the 10,000 steps down into bite-size chunks.

DAY 13

Today's mantra: *I've come a long way in 2 weeks!*
Today's step target: 10,000
Tip/testimony from volunteer: *I feel so proud of what I've achieved. I feel so much more active and I'm still keeping to the diet and exercise. I have bad days, but when I do, I just get back to the plan the next day instead of giving up.* **Tracy, 30**

On rising	1 glass of water plus cup of coffee, green tea or tea, or hot water and lemon
Suggested activity zone	15-minute walk (step target 1800)
Breakfast	2 glasses of water apricot and banana smoothie: soften 6 dried apricots in boiling water then place a ripe banana, a 4oz pot of natural yogurt, a spoonful of honey and ⅔ cup semi-skimmed milk into a blender, add the softened apricots and blend until smooth
Mid-morning spruce juice	choose a juice from those listed on page 14
Suggested activity zone	20-minute walk (step target 2400)
Lunch	1 glass of water a lunch from the options suggested on pages 71–9
Mid-afternoon snack	2 glasses of water a snack from the options listed on page 19

Suggested activity zone	30-minute walk (step target 3600)
Satisfying soup	1 bowl of FOG or Immune-boosting soup
Dinner	2 glasses of water a Starch Curfew meal from the selection on pages 80–97
Suggested activity zone	15–20-minute walk (step target 2200)
Bedtime drink	chamomile tea, hot milk or soya milk, or hot water and lemon

DEAR DIARY

Writing things down helps you keep track of what you're eating and also increases your awareness of your general diet and may draw your attention to shortfalls. For example, do you always feel tired mid-afternoon and succumb to a sugary snack? Do you always eat the same fruits and vegetables or do you include a wide variety of types? This information can help you shape a healthier diet. In addition, as you adopt healthier habits and reap the results, seeing it in black and white is very motivating.

DAY 14

Today's mantra: I am keen to continue with my new healthier lifestyle.

Today's step target: 10,000

Tip/testimony from volunteer: *Since starting this diet and exercise plan, I can't believe how much weight I've lost, how my body shape has changed and how much better I feel about myself. If everybody could have a Joanna Hall to advise and look after them I am sure the world would be a happier, slimmer and healthier place!* **Carol, 42**

On rising	1 glass of water plus cup of coffee, green tea or tea, or hot water and lemon
Suggested activity zone	15-minute walk (step target 1800) plus abdominal and core stability exercises (see page 22)
Breakfast	2 glasses of water breakfast grill: broil 3 tomatoes and a handful of mushrooms (sprayed with oil) and serve with 1 poached egg and a slice of wholewheat toast
Mid-morning spruce juice	choose a juice from those listed on page 14
Suggested activity zone	20-minute walk (step target 2400)
Lunch	1 glass of water a lunch from the options suggested on pages 71–9

Mid-afternoon snack	2 glasses of water a snack from the options listed on page 19
Suggested activity zone	30-minute walk (step target 3600)
Satisfying soup	1 bowl of FOG or Immune-boosting soup
Dinner	2 glasses of water a Starch Curfew meal from the selection on pages 80–97
Suggested activity zone	15–20-minute walk (step target 2200)
Bedtime drink	chamomile tea, hot milk or soya milk, or hot water and lemon

UPPING THE INTENSITY

If walking at a steady pace now feels like child's play, why not up the pace and try some intervals? Don't worry, you don't have to be an athlete to try interval training! Simply incorporate some faster bouts of power walking with your usual brisk pace. Use park benches, lampposts or even trash cans as markers to space out your intervals and make sure there's a marked difference between the pace of your fast bout and your recovery walk.

DAY 15

Congratulations on completing the 14-day plan. Chances are, you've lost weight, improved your fitness, and feel healthier. Here's how our volunteers got on, along with some of the positive changes they noticed:

Sharon, 26, lost 11lb and 4 inches
Natasha, 28, lost 2lb and 5½ inches
Melanie, 30, lost 4lb and 8 inches
Joan, 63, lost 6lb and 4.5 inches
Tom, 29, lost 6½lb and 4 inches
Tessa, 24, lost 5lb and 4 inches
Sam, 33, lost 4lb and 4 inches

- Clearer, brighter skin ☐
- Healthier, shinier hair ☐
- Improved digestion ☐
- More regular bowel movements ☐
- More energy ☐
- Less period pain or pre-menstrual tension ☐
- More positive outlook and greater self-confidence ☐
- Fewer headaches ☐
- Fewer colds and infections ☐
- Clearer thinking and improved mental function ☐

Why not check the boxes next to the benefit you have enjoyed on the Get a Grip plan?

QUICK FIXES

Remember to take your measurements again today (before you have eaten or drunk anything) to see how you have fared. If necessary, check page 30 to remind yourself how to take the measurements.

Now you should be ready for your big day or event—or simply feeling ready to take on the world. To maximize the results, we've provided a few final quick fixes to make you look and feel your best.

FREE FIXES

Stand tall: Hunched-over posture can add pounds to your frame. Stand tall by imagining you have a piece of thread running through your body and out of the crown of your head, which is gently pulling you upwards.
Pull it in: Being able to hold in your abdominals is a skill worth knowing. Don't suck everything in and hold your breath, though. Focus on mastering the rib–hip connection even when you are standing. Training your pelvic floor muscles will also help tone your lower abdominal muscles. To do this, take a breath into the lower rib cage and, as you exhale, draw up the muscles of the pelvic floor, as if you were trying to stop yourself having a pee.
Pile it up: Wearing your hair up adds height to your overall figure and makes your face look slimmer. If you

have short hair, try wearing it off your face to slim down features.

Go dark and mysterious: It's a fact—wearing black makes you look slimmer. If it drains your complexion, go for a dark color such as chocolate brown, eggplant or charcoal grey and wear the same color on top and bottom for a slimming effect.

CHEAP FIXES

Flush it out: Rid yourself of any excess fluid by drinking fennel or dandelion tea.

Disguise it: You can get some fantastically clever underwear these days, from tights and panties with tummy control panels to "butt-lifting" tights. Check out your local department store to see what's on offer.

TREAT FIXES

Get sun-kissed: A golden glow always gives a leaner look than pasty white skin. Treat yourself to a professionally applied fake tan. (If you're doing it at home, exfoliate first to prevent smears and patches.)

Wrap it up: Indulge in an Inch Loss Wrap. While this type of treatment won't provide lasting results, it will give you a 1–2 day inch loss as a result of fluid loss. It may be just the extra confidence kick you need for your big event …

Now turn to page 101 to find out how to maintain your success for life …

GET A GRIP LUNCHES

You can choose any lunch option from the lists below. Obviously where we are at lunchtime dictates what we can eat, so the lunch options are split into store-bought options, home options and packed lunches. All you have to do is choose …

Note: All of the lunch options can be served with unlimited vegetables or salad from the list on page 48.

STORE-BOUGHT LUNCH OPTIONS

- any store-bought sandwich under 350 calories
- any store-bought sushi under 350 calories
- any vegetable-based soup under 35 calories per ½ cup, plus a small bread roll and a piece of fruit

HOME OPTIONS

Baked Potato with Tuna

One small baked potato topped with 3½-oz can of tuna in brine or spring water mixed with some chopped red onion and cucumber and served on a bed of mixed salad leaves.

Info per serving:
Calories: 308.0
Fat: 1. 9g
Saturated Fat: 0.4g
Protein: 32.2g
Carbohydrate: 42.3g

Egg on Toast

One slice of rye toast, 2 boiled eggs with sliced broiled tomato and mushrooms brushed with olive oil and sprinkled with mixed herbs.

Info per serving:
Calories: 241.0
Fat: 12.9g
Saturated Fat: 3.0g
Protein: 11.8g
Carbohydrate: 19.5g

Tomato Soup

A bowl of fresh tomato soup (from the supermarket refrigerated section) topped with 2 tablespoons of cottage cheese, a handful of chopped cucumber and red pepper, and quarter of a chopped ripe avocado.

Info per serving:
Calories: 242
Fat: 8.0g
Saturated Fat: 1.0g
Protein: 14.2g
Carbohydrate: 23.0g

Beans on Toast

Two small slices rye bread, toasted, topped with a small can of baked beans (5oz) and ½ a 4oz pot of cottage cheese or a tablespoon of reduced-fat grated hard cheese.

Info per serving:
Calories: 296.0
Fat: 2.8g
Saturated Fat: 0.9g
Protein: 19.9g
Carbohydrate: 51.9g

The following lunch recipes serve more than 1 and can easily be broken down. Why not start the Get a Grip plan with a friend or neighbor and take it in turns to do the lunch? Support on your plan can really help your efforts.

Chicken and Corn Soup with Chili

Serves 4

4 cups chicken stock
2 chicken breasts, skinned and cubed
½-inch piece fresh root ginger, peeled and grated
½ small red chili, seeded and finely chopped (optional)
1 small can corn, drained and rinsed
1 bunch green onions, finely sliced diagonally
2 tablespoons soy sauce
salt and freshly ground black pepper
1 tablespoon fresh chopped cilantro

Info per serving:
Calories: 296.0
Fat: 2.8g
Saturated Fat: 0.9g
Protein: 19.9g
Carbohydrate: 51.9g

Put the stock into a large saucepan and bring to a boil. Add the chicken and poach until cooked through—about 5 minutes.

Add the ginger, chili and drained corn. Stir in the onions and simmer for 2 minutes. Season to taste, sprinkle in the cilantro and serve.

Joanna's top tip: You can get some great "home-made" style soups in the refrigerated section of your local supermarket. There are some very tasty chicken and corn versions—so if you are into convenience—add this to your weekly shopping list.

Roasted Butter Beans with Tomatoes

Serves 4

2 teaspoons olive oil
2 x 14-oz cans butter beans, drained and rinsed
4 ripe plum tomatoes, quartered
1 tablespoon sun-dried tomato paste
1½ tablespoons balsamic vinegar
good handful of fresh cilantro
salt and freshly ground black pepper

Info per serving:
Calories: 321.8
Fat: 10.9g
Saturated Fat: 1.3g
Protein: 15.2g
Carbohydrate: 42.1g

Preheat the oven to 200°C/400°F.

Heat the olive oil in a large roasting pan. Add the beans and tomatoes, stirring to coat them well with the oil. Season them with pepper only. Roast on the top shelf for 10 minutes, giving the pan a little shake halfway through.

Stir the tomato paste and vinegar into the beans and tomatoes and season to taste. Stir the cilantro in gently and serve with a slice of toasted whole-wheat bread or a small baked potato.

PACKED LUNCH OPTIONS

Soup with Bread and Cheese

One small thermos of Immune-boosting or Full of Goodness soup (see page 18 for recipes) with a small whole-wheat roll and 1oz Edam cheese.

Sandwich Options

Choose one of the following:	**Add one of the following fillings or toppings:**	**Pile on:**	**Season with:**
small pitta bread	tuna in brine	any salad or vegetable items from the unlimited list on page 48	grainy mustard
medium whole-grain roll	hard-boiled egg		tomato salsa
small bagel	chicken breast		mango chutney
slice of whole-wheat bread	flavored cottage cheese		reduced-fat tzatziki
	smoked salmon or canned pink salmon		natural yogurt
	lean sliced ham		
	prawns		
	grated Edam cheese		

White Bean and Tuna Salad

Serves 6

Info per serving:
Calories: 314.0
Fat: 6.4g
Saturated Fat: 0.9g
Protein: 32.3g
Carbohydrate: 31.0g

3½ cups fine green beans, topped and tailed and cut small
3 x 14-oz cans cannellini beans, drained and rinsed
1 red onion, finely diced
2 tablespoons wholegrain mustard
6 tablespoons white wine vinegar
⅛ cup olive oil
salt and freshly ground black pepper
good handful flat leaf parsley, roughly chopped
3 x 7-oz cans light meat tuna in brine, well drained
Bag of salad

Drop the green beans in boiling water and cook for 3–5 minutes until just cooked. Drain and rinse well in cold water. Put the cannellini beans into a bowl with the red onion. In another bowl, whisk together the mustard, vinegar and oil and season to taste. Mix into the beans and onion. Add the drained green beans and the parsley. Break the tuna up into big chunks and mix into the salad.

Joanna's top tip: This is a quick lunch to rustle up for friends—they will never know how healthy it is!

Shrimp and Cucumber Salad with a Minty Dressing

Serves 2–3

Info per serving:
Calories: 202.3
Fat: 11.8g
Saturated Fat: 1.7g
Protein: 18.5g
Carbohydrate: 5.2g

½ cucumber, halved lengthways and seeded using a teaspoon (cucumber seeds make any salad very watery)
6oz shelled cooked shrimp
1 tablespoon chopped mint
½ teaspoon sugar
1 tablespoon boiling water
1 tablespoon white wine vinegar
1 tablespoon olive oil
salt and freshly ground black pepper
romaine lettuce leaves to serve the shrimp in

Slice the cucumber halves into half moons and place in a bowl together with the shrimp. Place the mint and sugar in a bowl and pour over the boiling water. Leave for 5 minutes and then stir in the vinegar and oil and season well. Add the shrimp and cucumber and stir to coat well.

Arrange the lettuce on a serving plate and spoon the shrimp salad on top. Serve with a slice of whole-wheat bread or a baked potato.

Red Bean and Tomato Salsa Salad

Serves 2–3

15-oz can red kidney beans, drained
1⅓ cups tomatoes, finely chopped
½ red onion, finely chopped
rind of 1 lime, grated
juice of 2 limes
1 large ripe but firm avocado, peeled, stoned and diced
2 tablespoons olive oil
1 green chili, very finely chopped
good handful of fresh cilantro, finely chopped
salt and freshly ground black pepper

Info per serving:
Calories: 336.0
Fat: 19.9g
Saturated Fat: 2.8g
Protein: 10.2g
Carbohydrate: 34.9g

Put everything into a bowl and stir well. Chill until ready to eat.

Joanna's top tip: **Use rubber gloves when chopping the green chili or wash your hands well afterwards.**

Chicken and Sun-Dried Tomato Salad

Serves 4

4 cooked, skinned chicken breasts
2oz Black Forest ham, cut into strips and all traces of fat removed
2oz pine nuts, tossed into a hot, dry frying pan for a few seconds until golden
7-oz jar sun-dried tomatoes or sun-blush tomatoes, well drained and sliced
a handful of fresh basil leaves (optional)
bag of mixed salad leaves

Info per serving:
Calories: 300.0
Fat: 12.0g
Saturated Fat: 4.1g
Protein: 33.4g
Carbohydrate: 14.4g

For the dressing:
1 tablespoon balsamic vinegar
1 tablespoon olive oil or you can use the oil from the jar of tomatoes
½ teaspoon Dijon mustard
salt and freshly ground black pepper

Slice the chicken breasts diagonally and arrange on a serving plate. Scatter the ham over the top, followed by the tomatoes and the pine nuts. Whisk the dressing ingredients together and drizzle over the salad. Scatter the basil over the top and serve with mixed salad leaves.

GET A GRIP STARCH CURFEW DINNERS

All of the following meals follow my Starch Curfew principle, which means none of them includes starch—and of course they shouldn't be served with rice, potatoes, bread, pasta and so on. Instead of accompanying your meals with starch you will be filling up on vegetables, so get acquainted with the unlimited vegetables list page 48 and serve plenty with every meal. Not only will serving vegetables and salads instead of starch reduce your calorie intake, it will also make a good contribution to the minimum of five portions of fruit and vegetables you should be having each day.

You'll find more information on why my Starch Curfew is such a successful strategy on page 108.

MEAT-BASED DISHES

Quick Honey Pork Chops

Serves 4

2 tablespoons honey
1 tablespoon grated fresh root ginger
1 tablespoon soy sauce
1 garlic clove, crushed
4 pork chops

Info per serving:
Calories: 302.0
Fat: 12.7g
Saturated Fat: 5.0g
Protein: 35.6g
Carbohydrate: 9.7g

Preheat broiler to medium. Meanwhile, mix the honey, ginger, soy sauce and garlic together in a small bowl and set aside.

Broil the chops for 10 minutes, remove from the broiler, brush the glaze over the chops and cook for another 5 minutes.

Cheater's Spicy Fillet Steaks

Serves 2

9oz Ready to Cook Vegetable Selection
2 fillet steaks (approx 5oz each)
11-oz jar fresh vegetable-based pasta sauce such as spicy arrabbiata or napoletana
4 tablespoons red wine

Info per serving:
Calories: 303.0
Fat: 11.2g
Saturated Fat: 6.4g
Protein: 29.5g
Carbohydrate: 18.1g

Cook the vegetables as instructed on the package. Heat a lightly oiled pan or griddle and sear the steaks on each side for 4 minutes.

While the steaks are cooking, put the sauce in a pan with the wine and cook through, stirring well.

Place the steaks on warm plates with the vegetables, spoon the sauce around the steaks and serve.

Quick Chicken and Chickpea Curry

Serves 4

2 onions, thinly sliced
1 teaspoon light olive oil
2 tablespoons curry paste
2 cups chicken stock
14oz cooked chicken breast meat, chopped
14-oz can chickpeas, drained
2 x 14-oz cans lentils, drained

Info per serving:
Calories: 363.0
Fat: 3.0g
Saturated Fat: 2.2g
Protein: 40.9g
Carbohydrate: 42.5g

Soften the onion in the oil for 4–6 minutes. Stir in the curry paste and cook for 2 minutes.

Add the stock, chicken and chickpeas and stir well. Bring to a boil and cook, uncovered, for about 15 minutes until the chicken is hot and the sauce has reduced and thickened.

Heat the lentils through in the microwave and divide between each plate. Top with the curry and serve.

Quick Zucchini Bolognese

Serves 4

Info per serving:
Calories: 385.0
Fat: 24.5g
Saturated Fat: 9.4g
Protein: 25.6g
Carbohydrate: 19.1g

1 teaspoon olive oil
1 red pepper, seeded, cored and coarsely chopped
1lb lean minced pork
11-oz jar Arrabiata sauce (most supermarkets stock this)
sprinkling of freeze-dried parsley
8 zucchini, sliced lengthways with a potato peeler to make ribbons

Heat the oil in a pan, add the red pepper and cook for 3–4 minutes.

Add the pork and cook, stirring and breaking it up, until it starts to brown. Drain through a sieve to remove excess fat and return to the pan. Pour in the sauce and add two tablespoons of water. Partly cover the pan and cook for 15–20 minutes, stirring occasionally.

Meanwhile, cook the zucchini ribbons in a pan of boiling water for 3–4 minutes until just cooked, and then drain. Divide between the plates and top with the meat sauce.

Red Pesto Chicken with Cucumber Salad

Serves 4

4 skinned chicken breasts
olive oil
¾ cup low-fat crème fraiche
14-oz can chopped tomatoes
3 tablespoons red pesto (fresh or from a jar)
salt and freshly ground black pepper
fresh basil and black olives (optional)

Info per serving:
Calories: 321.3
Fat: 18.4g
Saturated Fat: 6.3g
Protein: 29.6g
Carbohydrate: 8.6g

For the cucumber salad:
½ cucumber, halved lengthways and seeded with a teaspoon
1 spring onion
Mitsukan seasoned rice wine vinegar (from any good supermarket)

Fry the chicken breasts in a little oil until browned. Remove from the frying pan and place in a large saucepan or stove-top casserole dish.

Combine the crème fraiche, tomatoes and pesto, season and pour over the chicken.

Cover the chicken and cook over a low heat for 40 minutes.

Meanwhile, thinly slice the halved cucumber together

with the onion and put in a bowl. Pour over 2 tablespoons seasoned rice wine vinegar and mix in well. Leave for 30 minutes to allow the flavors to develop.

Serve the chicken accompanied by the cucumber salad.

FISH DISHES

Best-Ever Caesar Salad

Serves 2

Info per serving:
Calories: 319.5
Fat: 29.5g
Saturated Fat: 4.3g
Protein: 7.9g
Carbohydrate: 8.4g

2 anchovy fillets
1 large garlic clove, crushed
1 teaspoon Dijon mustard
1 teaspoon red wine vinegar
¼ teaspoon Tabasco or any hot pepper sauce
¼ cup olive oil
1 large romaine lettuce, washed, drained and torn into bite-size pieces
1 tablespoon freshly grated Parmesan

Mash the anchovies with the back of a fork and put into a large bowl with the garlic, mustard, vinegar and pepper sauce. Mix well. Slowly drizzle in the olive oil, whisking all the time so it doesn't curdle.

Add the lettuce and cheese and toss together well. Add salmon, smoked salmon, flaked tuna or cold boiled eggs if desired.

Wrapped Salmon

Serves 2

Squeeze of lemon juice
4 skinless salmon fillets
4½oz prosciutto ham, all fat removed
1 package chives

Info per serving:
Calories: 338.0
Fat: 18.4g
Saturated Fat: 4.5g
Protein: 39.3g
Carbohydrate: 2.2g

Preheat the oven to 180°C/350°F.

Squeeze a little lemon juice over the salmon fillets and wrap two slices of ham around each piece of salmon. Place in an ovenproof dish and sprinkle with snipped chives. Bake in the oven for 8–10 minutes.

Broiled Salmon with Basil and Lemon Dressing

Serves 4

4 salmon fillets
4 teaspoons extra virgin olive oil
finely grated zest and juice of ½ lemon
1 garlic clove, crushed
small handful torn basil leaves

Info per serving:
Calories: 280.3
Fat: 18.2g
Saturated Fat: 3.5g
Protein: 26.7g
Carbohydrate: 0.9g

Preheat the broiler. Line the broiling pan with foil, lay the salmon fillets on top and broil for 5–6 minutes on each side. While they are cooking, whisk the olive oil, lemon zest and juice, garlic and basil together. Drizzle over each salmon fillet when serving.

Ratatouille and Tuna Frittata

Serves 4

2 x 14-oz cans ratatouille

14-oz can tuna in brine, well drained and flaked

olive oil spray

5 whole eggs

5 egg whites

½ cup Edam cheese, grated

salt and freshly ground black pepper

Info per serving:
Calories: 348.0
Fat: 13.0g
Saturated Fat: 6.5g
Protein: 38.7g
Carbohydrate: 14.4g

Drain most of the juice from the ratatouille.

Spray a large non-stick frying pan with olive oil and heat the pan. Add the ratatouille and flake the tuna over the top.

Beat the whole eggs and the egg whites together and season. Pour the eggs over the ratatouille and tuna. Cook over a gentle heat, lifting the edges occasionally until nearly cooked through.

Sprinkle the cheese over and finish off under a medium broiler.

Tuna Teriyaki with a Lettuce and Sweet Ginger Stir-Fry

Serves 4

Info per serving:
Calories: 262.0
Fat: 13.2g
Saturated Fat: 2.5g
Protein: 27.6g
Carbohydrate: 5.9g

4 x 4-oz tuna steaks
1 large romaine lettuce, washed and sliced at 1-inch intervals
1 tablespoon olive oil

For the marinade:
2 tablespoons Japanese soy sauce
2 tablespoons dry white wine
2 tablespoons Japanese rice vinegar or white wine vinegar

For the sauce:
1 tablespoon olive oil
2 large shallots, peeled and finely chopped
1-inch cube fresh root ginger, peeled and grated
1 large garlic clove, crushed
1 teaspoon dark, soft brown sugar
½ teaspoon sesame oil

Preheat oven to 220°C/425°F.

Combine the marinade ingredients and pour over the tuna steaks in a shallow dish, coating them well. Cover and set aside for 30 minutes. When time is up, remove the tuna from the marinade, reserving the marinade. Place the tuna on a baking sheet lined with foil and cook in the oven for 7–10 minutes.

Fry the shallots in a tablespoon of olive oil until golden. Add the ginger and garlic and continue to cook for a further minute. Add the reserved marinade and the sugar and cook until the sugar begins to caramelize and the sauce is thick and glossy. Remove from the heat and stir in the sesame oil.

Wok-fry the lettuce over a high heat in a tablespoon of olive oil until it just begins to wilt. You may need to add a tablespoon of water or soy sauce to create some steam.

Serve the fish on top of the lettuce, with some sauce drizzled over.

VEGGIE DISHES

Crustless Vegetable and Pesto Quiche

Serves 4

1 teaspoon light olive oil
1 yellow and 1 orange pepper, seeded and quartered
2 zucchini, cut into chunks
2 red onions, cut into 8 wedges
4 large eggs, beaten
½ cup semi-skimmed milk
2 tablespoons pesto
salt and freshly ground black pepper

Info per serving:
Calories: 184.3
Fat: 9.6g
Saturated Fat: 1.9g
Protein: 10.8g
Carbohydrate: 15.9g

Preheat the oven to 200°C/400°F.

Heat the oil in a non-stick pan, add the vegetables and flash-fry on a high heat for 2–3minutes. Transfer the vegetables to an ovenproof quiche dish.

In a bowl, mix together the eggs, milk, pesto and seasoning. Pour over the vegetables and bake in the oven for 20–30 minutes until the center is just firm to the touch.

Spicy Chickpea Balls with Minty Yogurt Sauce

Serves 4

2 x 16-oz cans chickpeas, drained
3 garlic cloves, crushed
2 teaspoons ground cilantro
2 teaspoons ground cumin
2 tablespoons fresh chopped parsley
salt and freshly ground black pepper
olive oil for frying

Info per serving:
Calories: 187.6
Fat: 4.8g
Ssaturated Fat: 1.6g
Protein: 7.9g
Carbohydrate: 29.4g

For the sauce:
1⅓ cups natural yogurt
good handful of fresh chopped mint leaves
2 teaspoons lemon juice
salt and freshly ground black pepper

Place the chickpeas, garlic, cilantro, cumin and parsley in a blender or food processor and blend together. Season well and blend again until smooth.

Form the mixture into small patties.

Heat a little olive oil in a frying pan and fry the patties in small batches in the hot olive oil. Drain well on kitchen paper.

Combine all the ingredients for the sauce and chill.

Serve the patties with the sauce and a crisp green salad.

Flageolet Bean Casserole

Serves 4

1 teaspoon light olive oil
3 zucchini, cut into chunks
2 garlic cloves, crushed
150ml dry white wine
2 x 11-oz tubs fresh tomato pasta sauce
2 x 14-oz cans flageolet or navy beans, drained and rinsed
salt and freshly ground black pepper

Info per serving:
Calories: 281.8
Fat: 5.3g
Saturated Fat: 0.8g
Protein: 13.2g
Carbohydrate: 41.1g

Heat the oil in a large frying pan and fry the zucchini for 8 minutes over a medium–high heat, stirring often. Add the garlic when the zucchini is almost cooked. Add the wine and boil rapidly for 2 minutes to reduce by half. Add the tomato sauce and beans and simmer for 5 minutes. Season to taste.

Easy Piperade

Serves 3–4

A much tastier classic French version of scrambled eggs.

1 tablespoon olive oil
2 each of red, green and yellow peppers, cored, seeded and sliced into strips
1 red onion, thickly sliced
2 large garlic cloves, crushed
6–8 large beaten eggs
salt and freshly ground black pepper

Info per serving:
Calories: 230.0
Fat: 12.6g
Saturated Fat: 3.3g
Protein: 13.4g
Carbohydrate: 17.5g

Heat the oil in a non-stick wok or pan and fry the peppers and onion until they begin to soften but not brown. Add the garlic and cook for a further 2 minutes.

Season the eggs well and add them to the pan, stirring them into the vegetables gently until the egg is set. Check again for seasoning and enjoy, hot or cold!

Butter Bean, Olive, and Feta Salad

Serves 4

This is a good summer salad.

4 ripe tomatoes
1 tablespoon light olive oil
juice of 1 lemon
2 x 14-oz cans butter beans, drained
⅓ cup black olives
1 red onion, thinly sliced
2 cups feta, cubed

Info per serving:
Calories: 337.0
Fat: 11.5g
Saturated Fat: 6.5g
Protein: 18.2g
Carbohydrate: 35.6g

Chop one of the tomatoes and blend in a food processor or blender with the olive oil and lemon juice until fairly smooth.

Cut the remaining tomatoes into wedges and mix with the beans, olives, onion and feta.

Toss in the tomato dressing and serve.

SECTION 2

Well done, you've achieved your goal, you've dropped a size. Now it's all about …

HABIT BUILDING

HABIT-BUILDING STRATEGIES

So, it worked. Well, that's the first hurdle out the way. By now you should have lost some weight and be feeling fitter and healthier. But don't get complacent! Now, while you are feeling on top of things and the lessons of healthy eating and exercise are fresh in your mind, is the ideal time to make these strategies part of your everyday life. Remember, we had a deal—together we've proved that you *can* lose weight. You have done the Get a Grip plan. Now I want to show you how to *keep* it off. For lifelong results, there's no magic pill, just lots of small steps toward a healthier, fitter you. To help you understand these steps and help you make them part of your life, this section is divided into ten parts. Each part covers a proven strategy for successful weight control and a healthier you, with tips on how to implement it and why it works. Whether you implement all ten at once, or just address one or two a week, you'll be heading in the right direction. Come on, it's time to build some habits ...!

HABIT 1

MOVE MORE, MORE OFTEN

By now, you should have got the message that physical activity is an essential part of the weight-loss equation. Exercise boosts calorie-burning muscle mass, helps raise metabolic rate, and makes us feel good. Ask someone if they are physically active and most will remember how they've been running around all day and reply "yes". But think about it. OK, so you may feel "tired" at the end of each day but is it because you were *physically* active, *mentally* active, or *geographically* active? Here's an example: you wake up in the morning and think "today I have to take the kids to school, finish off that report, get the washing done, work half a day for my job, cook the dinner and do some homework for my evening class"—and that is just the first page on your To Do list. By the end of the day you are tired because you have had a *mentally* tiring day, having to juggle and complete so many tasks. But none of these has actually involved you moving your body very much. Let's look at another scenario: this time you have to take the kids to school, drop off the dry cleaning, take a package to the post office, pick up a prescription from the doctor, buy your food shopping from the supermarket, drop in to see a friend who has not been well, run downtown, stop by your office, pick up the kids at 4 p.m., take Johnny to soccer, Elizabeth to piano, the list goes on … All of these involve being in a different place, so you have been active but you have been *geographically* active—you have covered a great deal of distance but you have done it with a car, bus, or public transportation. You have been all over, traveled great distances but your body has barely moved at all.

So are you geographically active, mentally active, or are you actually physically active? One of the most important habits to try to build in this book is to *move your body more often*.

Many people say they haven't got time to be active. It can certainly feel that way sometimes, but think about this ... There are 24 hours in the day, and let's assume we sleep and rest for 9 hours—that leaves 15 hours when we are awake and could potentially be moving our bodies. Multiply that by 7 days a week and that leaves 105 hours a week available to us to move our bodies. Even if you go to the gym three times a week for 60 minutes, that leaves 102 hours of inactivity. So, as you can see, we are expecting a great deal of change in our weight and body-fat levels for our efforts, when effectively, we are only moving our bodies for a mere 3 hours a week. In fact, a study published in the journal *Nature* found that non-gym goers who were generally active in their daily lives (for example, walking instead of driving, doing manual tasks instead of paying other people to do them) were actually healthier and fitter than gym addicts who sweated it out three times a week but spent the rest of the time immersed in the convenience culture. So what about those other 165 hours? Move more, more often!

PUTTING THE MOVE MORE CONCEPT INTO PRACTICE

It's a really simple concept and it's free—it's about being creative with your available time to expend more energy without putting on your gym clothes. If you can navigate your day to find opportunities to move you body, you will find it makes a big impact on your daily calorie burn and your health.

WALK THIS WAY

It's been known for a long time that walking is good for our health, but the exciting thing is that we are now able to quantify this. Studies have shown that we need to walk a minimum of 4000 steps a day to achieve minimum health, 7000 steps a day can contribute to fitness, and 10,000 steps a day to weight loss. An hour's walk, five days a week, also helped women reduce their cholesterol levels significantly in a recent study. Taking 10,000 steps a day roughly equates to a calorie expenditure of 500 calories. If you manage this for seven consecutive days, that is equivalent to 3500 calories, which leaves you potentially 1lb of fat lighter. But the really good news is we can accumulate these steps right through the day. You don't have to do them all in one go. That is why in *Get a Grip* I tried to get you into the habit of taking walks throughout the day.

When I started the plan, I thought exercise was going to be a problem, as with two children, I never seem to have time to do anything for me. I take the children to school, go to work, pick the children up, take them dancing, swimming or to gymnastics, make their evening meal and then it's time for bed. When Joanna asked me to think about whether I was mentally active, geographically active or physically active, I realized that, although I'm constantly on the go, I am normally just driving from one place to another or sitting down for hours on end. I now swim while the children are dancing and walk while they're swimming. Now fitting in exercise isn't a problem at all. **Carol**

TAKE A MINUTE

If you have a desk-bound job, try to get up and move your body for 60 seconds every hour. In an average working day that could be an extra 8 minutes of exercise you are currently not doing. OK, it may not sound much, but if you did that five times a week that is an extra 40 minutes of physical activity that you are currently not doing. If you are able to move your body for 2 minutes each hour of the working day, that would equate to an extra 1 hour and 20 minutes of physical exercise—well worth the effort!

DON'T LABOR SAVE, LABOR SPEND!

We are surrounded by labor-saving devices and gadgets. You don't need to get up to switch TV channels, or answer the phone, you can stay in touch by email or cellphone—you don't have to do washing by hand or even put any effort into mashing potatoes! An American study recently reported that using email for 5 minutes out of every hour in your working day will cause a pound of weight gain a year—that's 10lb of surplus fat in the next decade!

All of this labor-saving is adding to our waistlines and undermining our health, so think of one labor-saving gadget you could do without and put it away—or even better, get rid of it all together. The list below provides some ideas.

ACCUMULATE ACTIVITY

You may now be a regular exerciser, but outside of your allocated training times you neglect your base physical-activity levels. Accumulating physical activity throughout the day has been shown to positively improve our health, and incorporating this consistently can have a big impact on the total energy we burn each day. Here are some ideas:

- Always walk up the stairs
- Leave your cellphone in the other room, so you have to move to answer it
- Think of something you do religiously each day (such as watch a favorite TV show or even brush your teeth!) and resolve to move your body for 5–10 minutes beforehand
- Walk for 10 minutes before buying lunch

- Walk up moving escalators
- Park the car at the farthest end of the parking lot
- Get off your bus a couple of stops before your usual stop and walk
- Resolve to always walk to mail a letter, buy a newspaper, etc.
- Increase your walking pace by 10 percent (see page 34)
- Walk an extra block to collect your lunch
- Walk to the next bus stop rather than the one nearest your home
- Don't email colleagues in the building—get up and talk to them
- When you are shopping, only use a cart if it's absolutely necessary. Otherwise carry it in a basket
- Do 10 squats or counter push-ups every time you are waiting for the coffee to brew
- Stand up on the train or bus rather than sitting

The great thing about physical activity is that it can be achieved without you having to put on your gym clothes. While there are certainly good reasons to do structured exercise (see point 3), if you get into the habit of being more physically active on a daily basis you will find it a great support strategy when life becomes a little too hectic to stick with your structured exercise sessions. Remember, our ancestors didn't have gyms and they were far fitter and slimmer than we are!

HABIT 2

OPERATE THE STARCH CURFEW

When you started the *Get a Grip* plan, you may have found the Starch Curfew, which effectively limits carbohydrate intake, a surprising strategy. After all, we've been told for years that carbohydrate is the nutrient of choice when it comes to health and weight control. But think about it: if the low-fat, high-carbohydrate diet was the solution, obesity levels would surely have fallen, not risen, over the last couple of decades. The problem is, we've come to believe that as long as we don't *eat* fat, we won't *get* fat—and that simply isn't the case. Too much of the wrong type of carbohydrate plays havoc with metabolism and blood sugar levels, which consequently affects satiety. Dr Walter Willett, chair of the department of nutrition at the Harvard School of Public Health, points out that we shouldn't be thinking of cutting out carbohydrates but simply being more choosy about the type of carbohydrate we eat. Initially, this can feel like a difficult strategy to take on. After all, most of us are accustomed to eating pasta, potatoes, or rice with our evening meal. But if you're anything like our volunteers, you probably found that not only did you get used to starch-free dinners but you also lost weight, gained energy, and didn't feel hungry. To understand how Starch Curfew works, you need to know a little about what happens when you eat carbohydrates. When we eat, carbohydrates are broken down to small useable units of glucose. First, glucose is released into the bloodstream, signaling the pancreas to produce the hormone insulin. Insulin takes some of the glucose to cells to give them immediate energy. It changes the rest of the glucose into a substance called glycogen, which is transported to the liver and muscles for short-term storage and then converted to fat if it is not needed.

This process works well when blood sugar is released slowly into the bloodstream, but if you eat the kind of carbohydrates that quickly convert to glucose, a high concentration of insulin is released. This causes blood sugar to drop suddenly, causing fatigue and cravings for more carbohydrates. The speed with which a carbohydrate causes a rise in blood sugar is measured by the Glycemic Index. The Glycemic Index ranks foods between 1 and 100 dependent upon their effect on raising blood sugar levels. The higher a food's GI rating, the faster blood sugar levels are raised and released into the bloodstream. Low GI foods, such as legumes, release sugar slowly into the bloodstream, keeping you satisfied for longer and preventing energy highs and lows. All of which helps you to stop craving sweet sugary snacks and keep hunger pangs at bay. The slower digestion and the more gradual rise and fall in blood sugar levels resulting from eating low glycemic index foods make them a healthier choice. A study from Harvard University's School of Public Health found that low-GI diets are associated with a lower

Low GI 50 or under	Moderate GI 50–70	High GI 70 and over
Yogurt	Brown rice	White rice
Lentils	Banana	Pasta (all types)
Apples	Corn	Cornflakes
Kelloggs All-Bran	Cous Cous	White bread
		Shredded wheat
Oatmeal	Honey	and Weetabix
Butter beans,	Sweet potato	Bagel
kidney beans		Parsnips, carrots,
Chick peas	Stoneground	baked potato
	wholewheat bread	Sports drinks
Milk	Crackers	French Fries
Dried apricots	Raisins	Watermelon

risk of Type II diabetes and heart disease, while Australian scientists are so convinced of the importance of the glycemic index that they have persuaded the government to include it on food labels. A healthy diet doesn't mean *only* eating low-GI foods, as many other factors (such as the amount of the food you eat, the amount of protein and fat you eat with it and the presence of fiber) also influence your overall blood sugar response. But try to include more low-GI foods in your diet and fewer high-GI foods and you'll soon see and feel a big difference in your energy levels. And by operating Starch Curfew, you'll see and feel a big difference in how your clothes fit. Use the chart opposite to help you get the right balance.

Most people know that the disease diabetes involves too much sugar in the blood and either not enough insulin to deal with it, or a failure in the insulin's ability to remove it. But did you know that, as we get older, insulin sensitivity decreases even in people who don't have diabetes? There is some evidence that suggests that if you eat a lot of high glycemic index carbohydrate foods, you become insensitive (or "resistant") to insulin and your body has to keep pumping out insulin, which, instead of converting the glucose into energy, turns it into fat. The various effects of this insulin resistance—"below-the-belt" fat accumulation, high concentration of blood fats, high blood pressure, and an increased risk of heart disease—have been termed Syndrome X. Developing the starch curfew habit helps you control your insulin levels, which in turn helps you stabilize your energy levels and reduce the risk of potential health problems.

You may be wondering if, with all the pitfalls of eating the wrong types of carbohydrate, it might be better just to stick with protein. The answer is no! High protein and very low carbohydrate diets aim to put the body in a state of ketosis. Ketosis means the body burns protein instead of carbohydrate for fuel. This approach is not supported by mainstream medical and nutritional establishment—in fact, the American Heart Association has actually put out a position statement condemning a high intake of protein as it increases blood cholesterol associated with heart disease and kidney disease. Starch Curfew allows you to apply a moderate approach to your eating, getting the balance right to fuel your energy and help you lose weight.

Following Starch Curfew has three benefits:

1. It cuts down calories without the calorie counting

By cutting out bread, pasta, rice, potatoes, and cereal after 5 p.m. you will naturally be cutting down your calories. But since you'll be filling up on more fruit and vegetables, lean meat, fish and slow-releasing energy-providing legumes, you won't feel hungry.

2. It boosts your energy

The starch curfew helps you get a better balance of nutrients. You will be eating more slow-releasing carbohydrates, which directly impact your energy levels and keep them steady. As you will be eating more fruit and vegetables, you will boost your intake of essential vitamins and minerals. You may think you already eat enough fruit and vegetables, but have a read of Richard's situation:

Before I discovered Starch Curfew I was convinced I was eating enough fruit and vegetables—I'd have muesli and toast for breakfast, a tuna and lettuce sandwich at lunch and an apple in the afternoon—though more often than not it was an apple Danish (well, that was a fruit, wasn't it?) and then pasta or risotto with a bit of salad or broccoli when I got home. My wife is an excellent cook, so I thought the fruit in my muesli and the lettuce leaf in my sandwhich, and maybe the token few peas in my risotto was enough! I actually discovered I was only hitting an average of two of my five suggested servings of fruit and vegetables a day. I knew about the link between fruit and vegetable intake and cancer—but I was sure I was fine! Once I started the Starch Curfew not only did I lose weight and feel fuller but I actually increased the amount of fruit and vegetables I ate without having to try too hard. It's so simple; it really worked for me. My wife does not have to cook me a different meal—it fits in with the rest of my family and I find it really effective as a businessman having so many lunches and dinners out. **Richard 46, who lost 5 inches off his waist and dropped 10lb**

To see what makes a portion of fruit or vegetables, check out the list below.

Salad, vegetables and fruit—what makes one serving?

- 10 asparagus spears
- 3 spears of broccoli or cauliflower
- 8 Brussels sprouts
- 3 sticks of celery
- half a zucchini
- 1 large tomato
- half a cucumber
- 1 small avocado

- medium bowl of lettuce
- 1 apple, orange, banana, pear, peach
- 1 large slice of melon, pineapple
- 4 dried apricots
- 1 cup berries

3. It reduces bloating

Excess starch intake can leave you feeling heavy and bloated. It's not surprising, when you understand that for every unit of glycogen (the storage form that carbohydrate takes in the body), you need to have 3 units of water with which to store it. Think of it this way—if you eat a cereal-bowl serving of pasta, your body has to hold on to three bowls of water to be able to convert the starch to glycogen to be stored. That's not to say we don't need glycogen—it is an essential fuel—but since we can only store a limited amount, if we are not burning it through regular exercise, it will be converted and stored as fat.

Refraining from eating carbohydrates after 5 o'clock has made an enormous difference to my life. I can hardly believe it. I no longer wake up in the middle of the night with a feeling of bloatedness and discomfort in my stomach, my digestion has improved and I feel so much better in myself. Starch curfew is not a diet, it's a lifestyle—I have never found an eating plan that so well suits my age group. I no longer suffer mood swings, I have loads more energy and I have really lost inches. My husband cannot believe it. I felt so much better that I told all my friends and they have felt the same, too. **Vanessa, 55 (lost 6 inches)**

PUTTING STARCH CURFEW INTO PRACTICE

Here are some tips to help you.

VEGGIE UP

Think fresh, frozen, and canned vegetables. Religiously walk down the fruit and vegetable aisles and fill that shopping cart—whether it's fresh, frozen, or canned fruit and vegetables, they all have their place!

At first, I was afraid my shopping budget would increase with buying all that fruit and vegetables. I'm a single mom, so for me every penny counts, even though I was really eager to get back in shape after the birth of my daughter. I found by following the starch curfew I had more energy—I stopped buying so many cookies and fillers to have in the afternoon to keep my energy levels up and my shopping bill actually went down, week in, week out—which was great! I even had some pennies to buy myself some clothes to celebrate all the inches I lost! **Emmaline, 28**

KEEP YOUR FINGER ON THE PULSE

If your idea of salad is a few lettuce leaves and a slice of tomato, think again. Salads can be spiced up with all kinds of things, from pine nuts and pumpkin seeds to finely chopped chilies, broiled mushrooms, sun-dried tomatoes, red kidney beans ... Be adventurous!

I'm so much more imaginative now with my salads—they become a meal in their own right, that way I do not feel deprived. I really like to steam vegetables and add them to mixed salad leaves. One of my favorites is to steam broccoli, asparagus, and snowpeas, run them under cold water to stop them overcooking, and throw in a big bag of salad leaves. I then dry-fry two big handfuls of button mushrooms in a little Thai sweet chili sauce and stir through the cooked and raw salad—it's really tasty, so simple and quick.
Carol, 44 (lost 10lb)

TRICK YOURSELF

If you feel a plate of dinner just doesn't look right without a heap of rice, pasta or potatoes, kid yourself by getting creative with presentation. Try cutting stir-fried zucchini into ribbons and laying your meat or fish on top of that, or purée or mash vegetables as if they were potato. For more ideas see the recipe for Quick Zucchini Bolognese on page 84.

HABIT 3

TAKE STRUCTURED EXERCISE

As you have now learned, exercise doesn't have to involve a pair of fancy sneakers and an expensive gym membership. In *Move More, More Often* (page 102) there are plenty of ideas about fitting more daily activity into your life. But for optimum weight-loss results, your best body shape and improved fitness, the ideal is to combine daily physical activity with regular structured exercise sessions. Health authorities recommend that to maintain health, we exercise at a low-to-moderate intensity for half an hour on most days of the week. For fitness gains, the intensity needs to be higher, which is why the American College of Sports Medicine recommends exercising more vigorously for 20–50 minutes, at least twice a week, alongside the more moderate activity. You should be working at a level that is intense enough to make you feel breathless and hot. Anything from step aerobics to salsa dancing counts! Here's how thrice-weekly sessions of your favorite activity can add up to some serious calorie expenditure …

Structured exercise to burn 1000 calories

3 x 45 minutes' in-line skating

3 x 40 minutes' jogging (12-minute miles)

3 x 40 minutes' bike-riding

3 x 1 hour 20 minutes' brisk walking

3 x 1 hour low-impact aerobics

3 x 40 minutes' tennis

PUTTING STRUCTURED EXERCISE INTO PRACTICE

- Pick an activity that you enjoy, not the one you think will burn the most calories.
- Sign up for a beginner's course in a dance class or sports activity—that way, you'll feel less intimidated and you'll be at the same level as everyone else.
- Write your workout dates and times in your diary as if they were an appointment, so that you don't end up crowding them out of your schedule.
- Be prepared—if your gym clothes are clean and packed, you'll be much more likely to go for a workout than if you have to hunt through the laundry basket for something to wear.
- Go with a friend. Not only does it provide moral support it also reduces the risk of you bailing out, as you'll be letting your friend down, too.

MUSCLING IN

Aerobic exercise—such as walking, jogging, or swimming—is the most important type of activity for your health, but resistance, or strength, training also plays a key role in weight control and in determining your body shape. Basal metabolic rate—the rate at which we burn calories at rest—begins to decline from 25–30 years of age, along with the volume of lean muscle tissue that we have. The result is an overall loss in metabolically-active tissue and a gain in highly inactive adipose—or fatty—tissue. One pound of muscle requires approximately 35 calories per day simply to function, while a pound of fat needs just one or two calories. So you can see that by increasing lean body mass through resistance training, this depressing shift in body composition can be reversed. An American study found that 12 weeks of regular resistance training resulted in a loss of 4lb of body fat and a gain of 3lb of lean muscle tissue. With regular practice, not only will you become a more efficient calorie-burning machine, you'll also look more toned, shapely, and firm. You don't have to join a gym to do resistance training—you can use your own body weight as resistance, or use dumbbells or household items, such as cans or water bottles, at home. Why not get started by following the Total Body Solution workout on page 120?

THE TOTAL BODY SOLUTION

This 15-minute workout blitzes the whole body—helping you to streamline muscles, tone up, and boost your metabolic rate by increasing your lean muscle mass. Each of the six exercises will provide two great benefits in one simple move. Ideally, I'd love you to complete the Total Body workout on non-consecutive days e.g. Tuesday, Thursday, Saturday, Monday—that way your body gets a chance to rest, you are not exercising all the time, and you get better results in the long-term. The workouts below cater for different levels so you can progress as your fitness and body tone increase. Remember to start out slowly, as studies have shown if you are too gung ho, motivation can quickly wane. If you think you can commit to doing the workout three times a week—that is great, but you need to be 90 percent confident you will be able to complete it three times. If not—let's aim for twice and appreciate the fact that you have made time in your busy day to do it—congratulate yourself for that and feel good about it, not bad that you have not been able to do three.

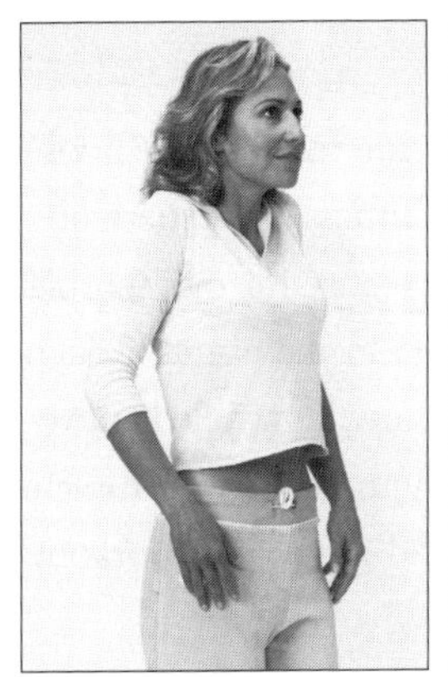

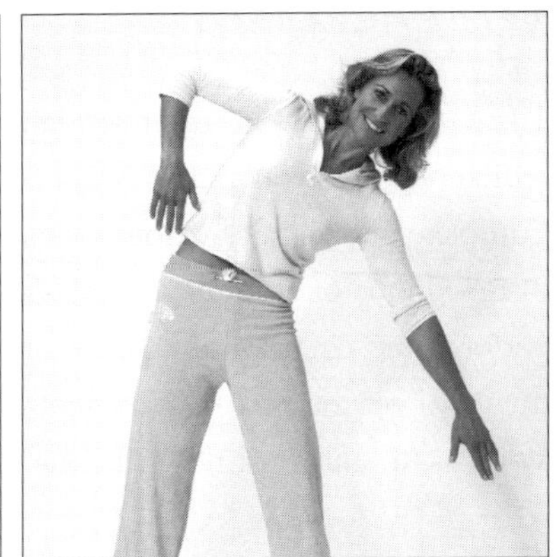

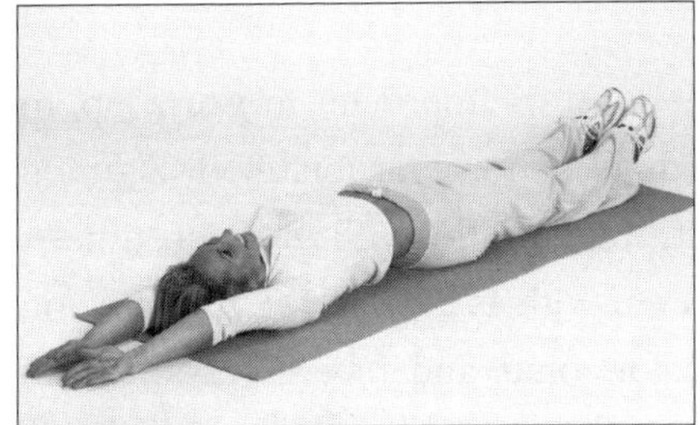

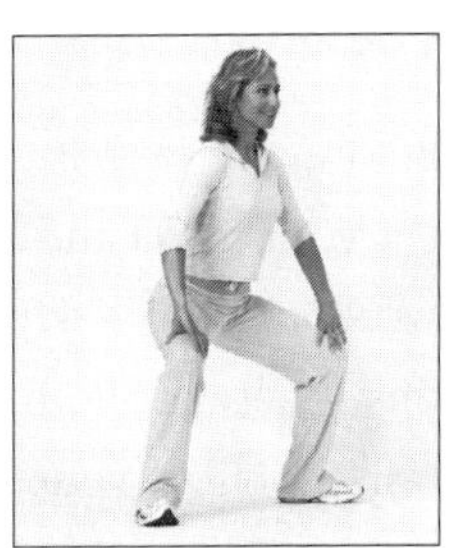

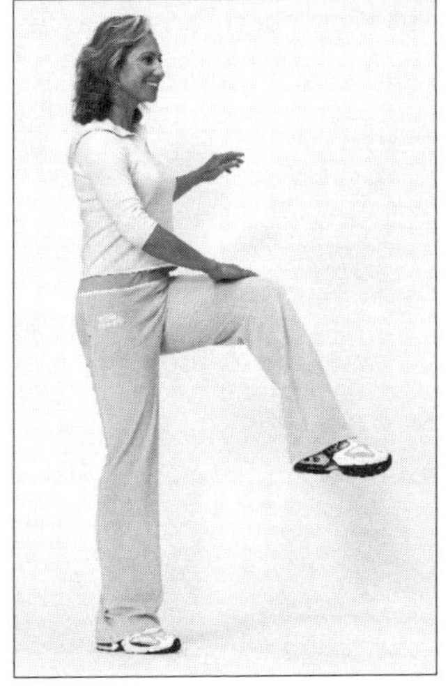

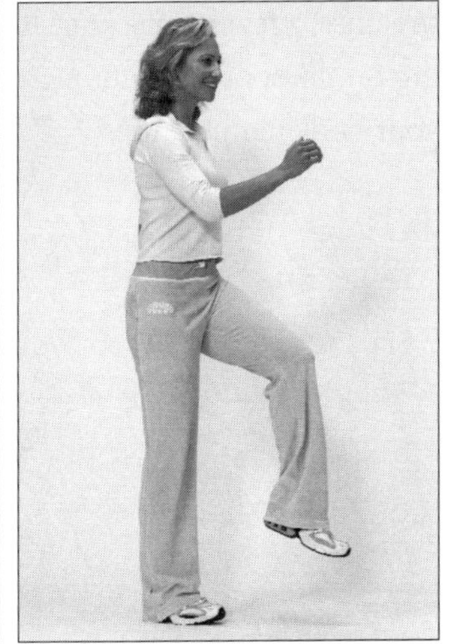

THE EXERCISES

There are two levels, beginners and intermediates. Choose which one suits you and your level of fitness and experience. Complete one circuit by doing each exercise for the number of repetitions or amount of time stated in the exercise. Then perform the circuit again. Focus on slow, controlled movements to get the best body benefits. Remember to complete a warm up and cool down before and after your workout.

WARMING UP

Before any exercise session it is important to warm up, to get your mind and body ready for your Total Body Solution workout. Don't skip it, thinking this will save you time—this is false economy. Even with as little as 3–5 minutes you can mobilize your major joints and relieve tension from your day—try shoulder rolls, some side bends and full body stretches, a few squats, knee lifts to your chest, brisk marching on the spot and running up and down stairs to increase your body temperature.

LEVEL ONE

Start with this workout if you are new to exercise or have had a break—you can always move on to level two if you feel it was too easy for you. Focus on good form and avoid rushing the exercises.

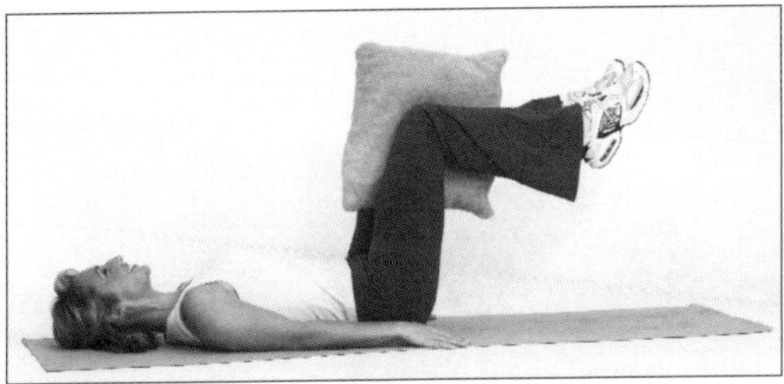

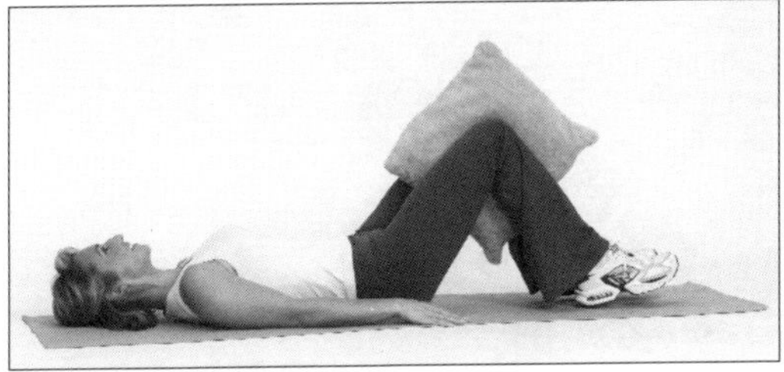

Body part: Torso

The exercise: Double leg drops

What it does: Flattens the abdominals

Extra Body part solution: Tones inner thighs

Lie on your back with a cushion between your legs, knees over chest. Keep your abdominals contracted and spine in a neutral position as you drop your legs to the floor so your toes lightly touch it. Continue for 60 seconds.

> *Joanna's top tip:* Remember to check out the rib–hip connection on page 23 of *Get a Grip* to help you with your technique.

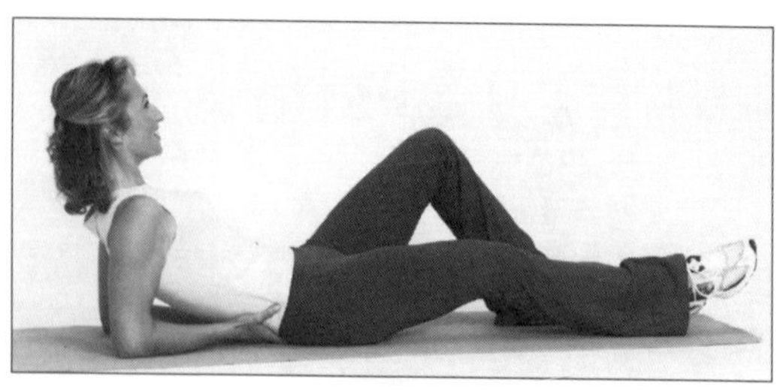

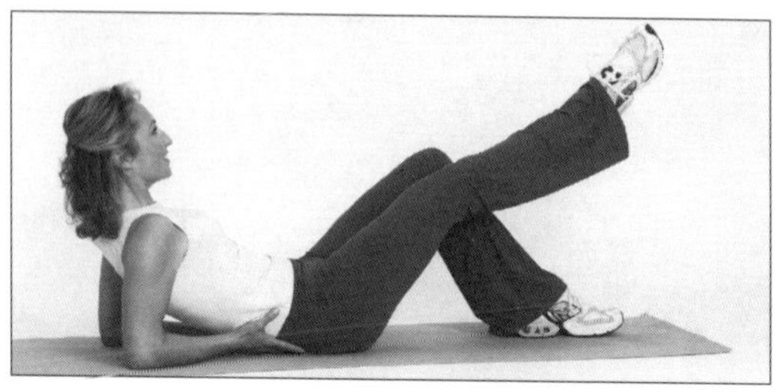

Body part: Legs

The exercise: Inner thigh lift with leg press

What it does: Tones inner thighs

Extra Body part solution: Streamlines whole thigh and helps strengthen weak knees

Lie on your back supported on your elbows, one leg straight and rotated out at the hip, the other leg bent. Soften the straight leg at the knee and lift it level to the height of the other knee, then lower. Lead from the inner thigh. Repeat 8 times and then hold the leg up and bring the ankle of the working leg into the knee and press away again. Repeat 8 times.

> *Joanna's top tip:* Keep the foot of the extended leg relaxed—this is important as it helps target the inner thigh muscles more.

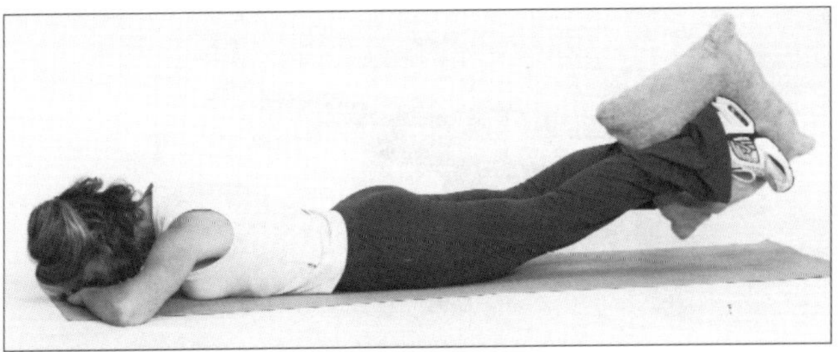

Body part: Butt

The exercise: Prone cushion lift

What it does: Tightens buttocks

Extra Body part solution: Stabilizes your spine and tones your abdominals

Lie face-down and place a small cushion between your ankles. Rest your forehead on your hands and pull in your abdominals to support your spine. Extend your legs and press the whole of the inner legs together as you squeeze the cushion between your ankles. Slowly and smoothly, lift your feet and legs about 6 inches off the floor and then slowly lower them to the ground. Continue for 60 seconds.

> *Joanna's top tip:* Make sure you extend your legs as long as possible as you lift them up off the floor. This helps to stabilize and build a strong spine and contract your buttock muscles more effectively.

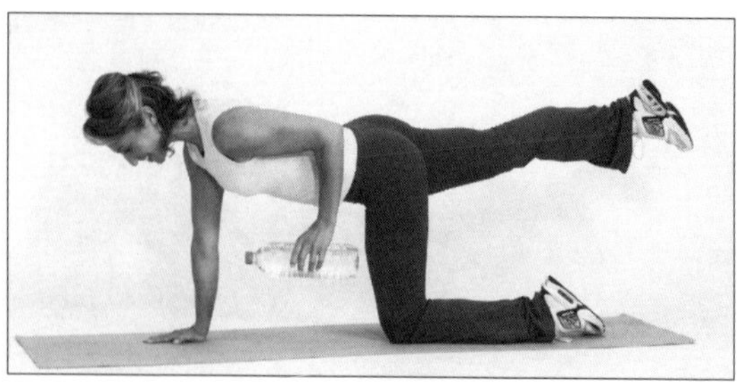

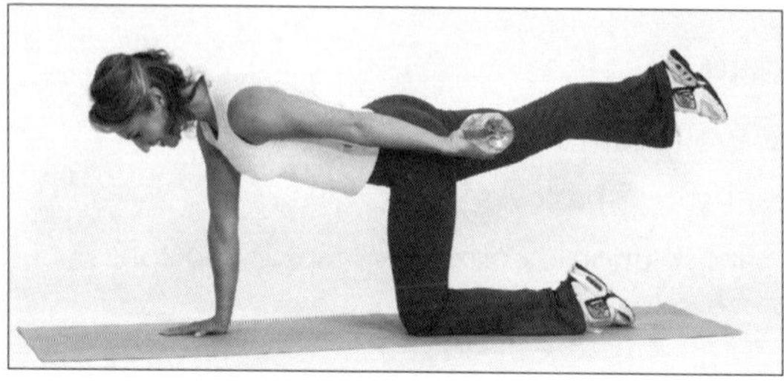

Body part: Chest and arms

The exercise: Kneeling triceps kickback

What it does: Streamlines backs of arms and tones trunk muscles

Extra Body part solution: Streamlines torso

On all fours, extend your left leg straight behind you. Keep abdominals contracted as you maintain a neutral spine. Hold a 2–3 liter weight in your right hand (or a large bottle of water) and hold your elbow close to your side, palm facing the mid-line of your body. Keep your elbow fixed as you extend your elbow back in line with your body. Rotate your palm toward the ceiling as you straighten your arm. Continue for 60 seconds, alternating arms and legs.

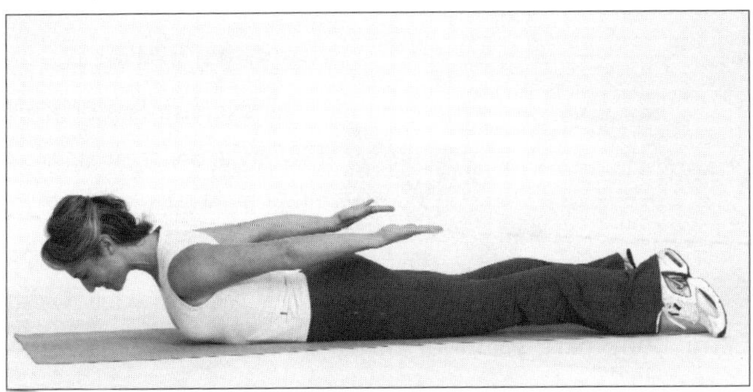

Body part: Back

The exercise: Back extension with arm lift

What it does: Tones and strengthens back

Extra Body part solution: Streamlines back of arms

Lie face-down, fingers resting by your side. Keep your abdominals contracted as you slowly lift your upper body off the floor. Keep your eye line down. Slowly lift your arms straight up, reaching your fingers to your feet. Lower your arms and then lower your upper body down to the floor. Continue for 60 seconds.

Joanna's top tip: **If you find this exercise too challenging, build up to it by keeping your hands on the floor.**

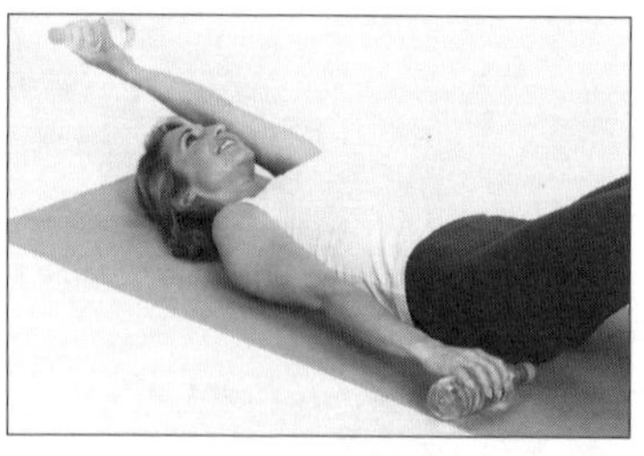

Body part: Arms

The exercise: Scissor arms

What it does: Streamlines the troublesome back of the arm area and helps you reclaim your waist!

Extra Body part solution: Helps draw the ribs together—particularly important post-pregnancy

Lie on your back, arms extended directly over your eye line. Hold one small weight—such as a can of tomatoes, a 4lb hand weight, or water bottle—in each hand. Slowly take four counts to lower your arms in opposite directions, one back over your head and the other toward your thighs. Keep your weight off the floor, lengthen through the arm as you lower it and keep your wrists in a neutral position. Draw the arms back over your eye line and scissor in the other direction. Do 8 full-range movements and then hold one arm level with your ears and lift about 2 inches slowly up and down 8 times. Repeat on the other side.

Joanna's top tip: This is a very subtle exercise but if you get the technique right it really tones the back of the arm. Avoid gripping the weight too tightly as this takes the emphasis away from the targeted muscle.

LEVEL TWO

This is a more challenging level—when you start out, why not try to complete just one set of 60 seconds of each exercise for three weeks and then progress on to two sets of 60 seconds?

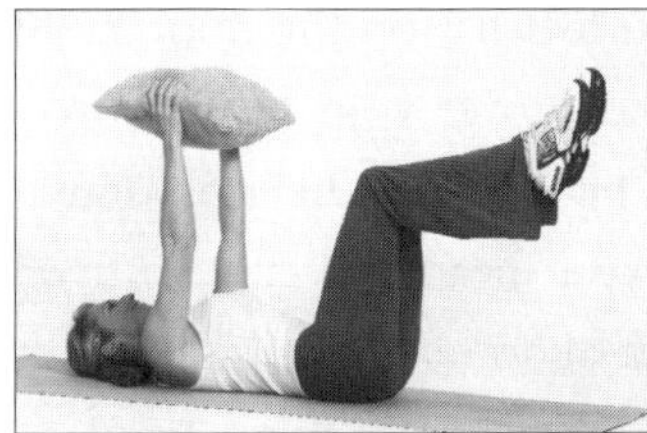

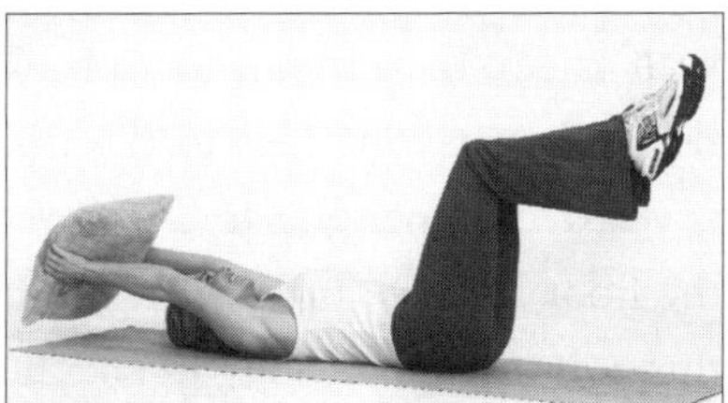

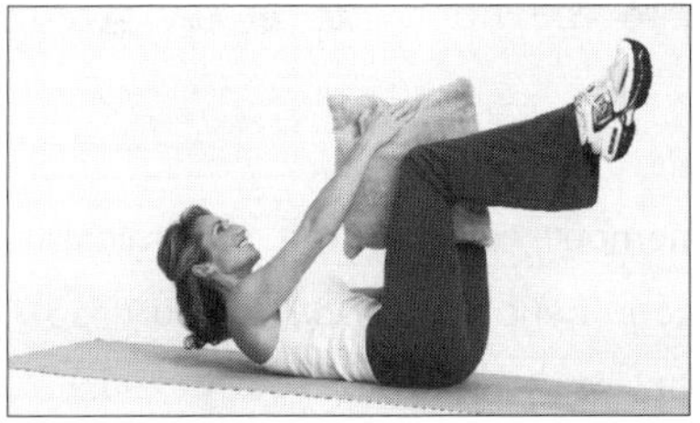

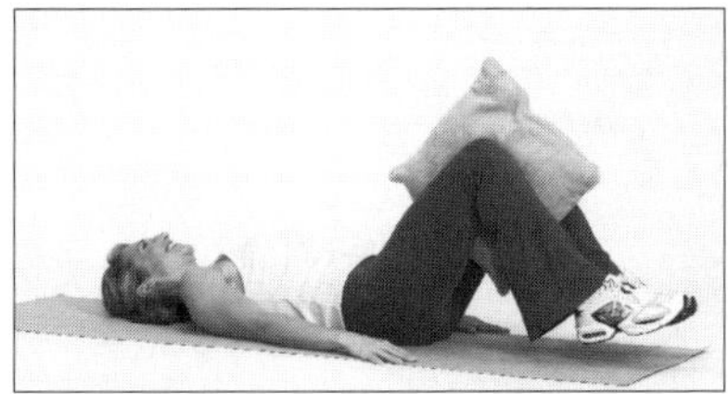

Body part: Abdominals

The exercise: Ab combo

What it does: Flattens abdominals, lengthens torso, and increases mobility of spine and shoulders

Extra Body part solution: Targets the legs as well as flattening whole of abdominal area and streamlining midriff

Lie on your back, knees bent, feet flat on the floor. Hold a cushion in your hands directly over your head. Slowly lower your arms over your head. Keep the ribs drawn in. Lift your arms back over your head and curl up from the breastbone to perform an abdominal curl as you lift your legs off the floor. Now place the cushion between your knees. Lower your torso back down to the floor and slowly lower your toes to the floor. Imagine the floor is covered in superglue to avoid you resting your feet on the floor. Draw your legs back into your chest, curling up through the upper body to take hold of the cushion once again. Lower your legs to the floor. Repeat the whole sequence.

> *Joanna's top tip:* Remember to keep the abdominals contracted and the spine in neutral position as you drop your legs to the floor, so your toes lightly touch.

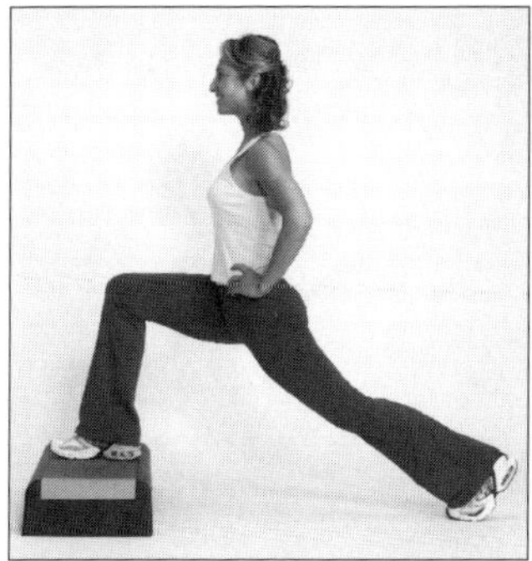
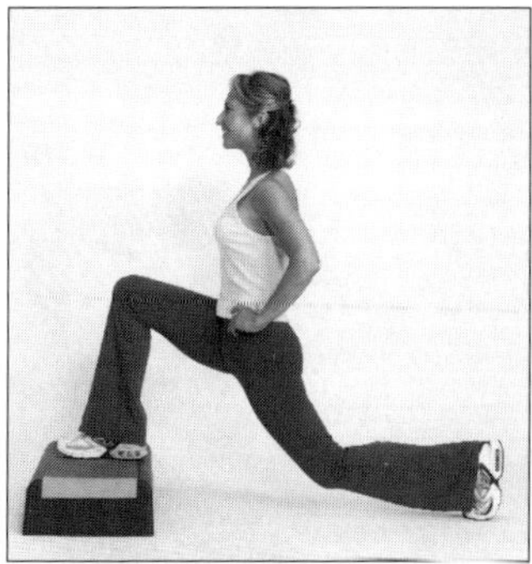

Body part: Legs

The exercise: Four point lunge

What it does: Shapes and strengthens thighs and gluteals

Extra Body part solution: The large number of muscles used in this exercise burns extra calories

Stand on a low bench or bottom stair. Extend one leg back with a large stride so the leg has only a slight bend at the knee, lower the knee of the extended leg towards the floor, straighten the leg and bring the extended leg back to the start position. Change sides.

> *Joanna's top tip:* Check the front knee is over your ankle, not your toe. Also check the knee is not rolling in—if you draw an imaginary line down your knee cap and through to your foot it should be in line with your second toe. Don't be afraid to use a chair for extra balance. It's much better to perform the exercise with good technique.

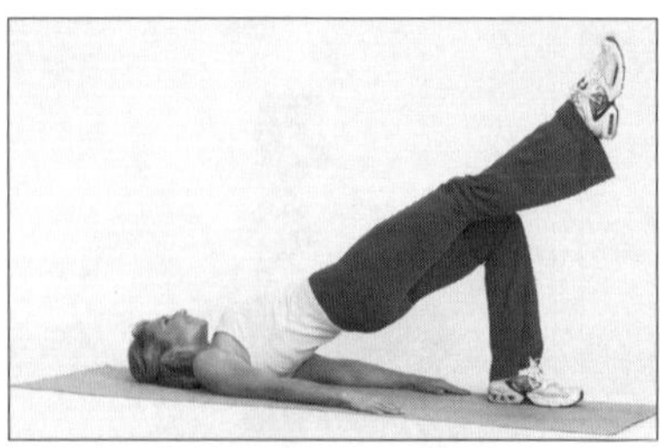

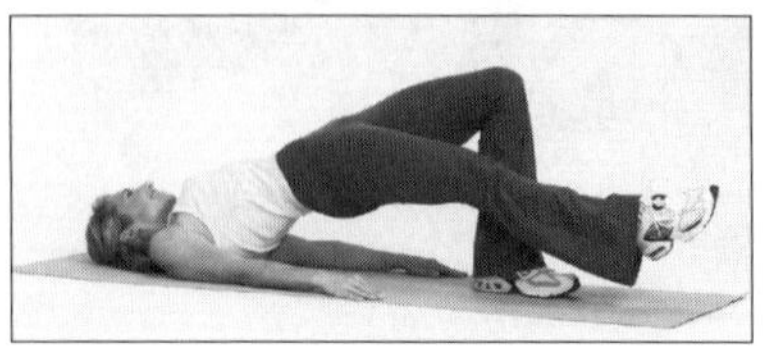

Body part: Buttocks

The exercise: Ab bridge with leg lift

What it does: Tightens buttocks, strengthens pelvic stabilizers

Extra Body part solution: Flattens abdominals and helps strengthen deep core trunk muscles important to your posture

Lie on your back, your knees bent at 90 degrees and your feet under your knees. Contracting your abdominals, tilt your pelvis as you peel off the floor, raising your body onto your shoulders, pushing your hips high. Keep your hips level and abdominals contracted to support your spine. Lift one leg straight and lift and lower it to the floor four times, contracting your buttocks as you lift. Take both feet flat to the floor and repeat on the other side.

> *Joanna's top tip:* This is a challenging exercise; make sure you do not drop your hips as you lift your leg. Pressing your knees away from your head will help you.

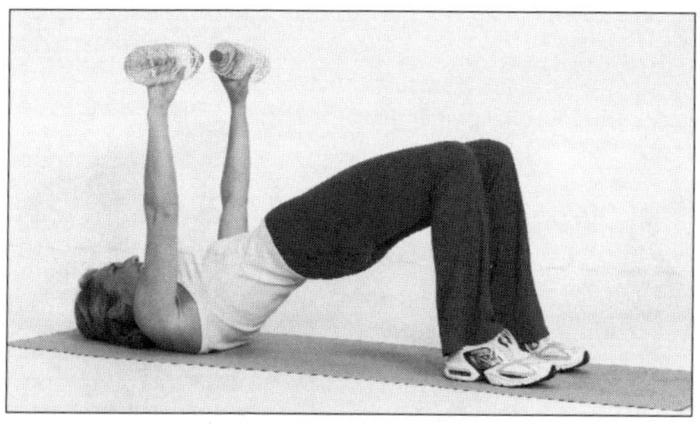

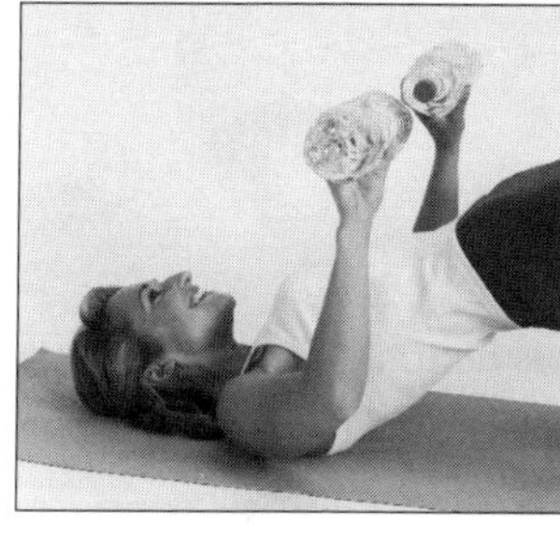

Body part: Chest

The exercise: Ab Bridge with chest press

What it does: Shapes shoulders and pectorals

Extra Body part solution: Tightens gluteals and hamstrings

Lying on your back with knees bent and feet flat on the floor, hold a dumbbell (or a large bottle of water) in each hand, with elbows bent at shoulder level. Tighten your buttocks and abdominals as you lift your buttocks off the floor into a bridge position. With your hips raised, press water bottles up over chest and then lower to start position. Maintain bridge and repeat chest press.

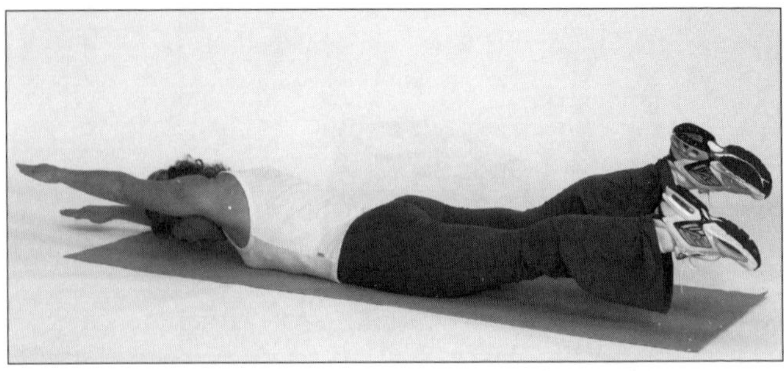

Body part: Back

The exercise: Swimming

What it does: Tones the back muscles

Extra Body part solution: Streamlines buttocks, thighs and arms

Lie face-down on the floor with your abdominals contracted. Lift your arms and legs and kick them as if swimming. Keep your body lengthened as you do this and your head in line with your spine.

> *Joanna's top tip:* Imagine you are trying to reach something with your feet and fingertips. Start slowly with this exercise until you have perfected the technique.

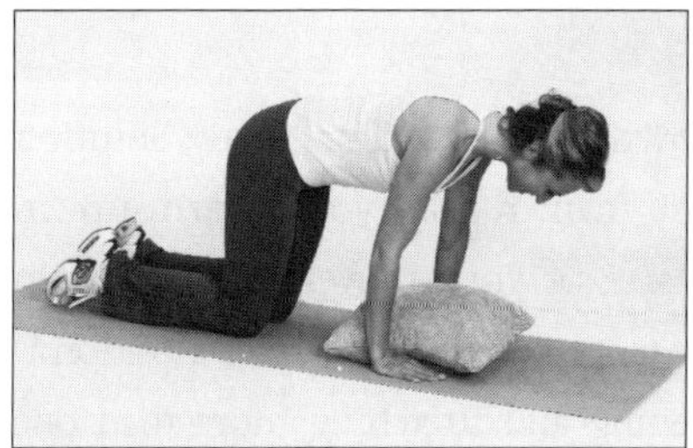

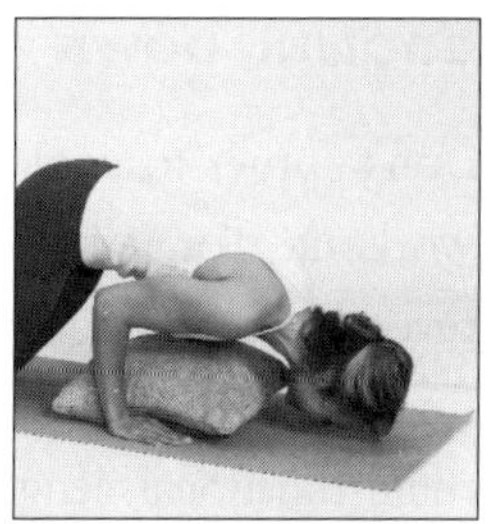

Body part: Arms

The exercise: Cushion press-up

What it does: Targets backs of arms

Extra Body part solution: Deep stabilization of the abdominals means you get a tummy workout as well

Come into a box position, wrists under shoulders and knees under hips. Place a cushion between your hands with your hands positioned mid-way at the side of the cushion. Draw your elbows back so they are by your sides. Draw your body forward so your face is over the front of the cushion. Slowly lower your upper body down to the floor with your nose in front of the cushion. You will feel a tightening at the back of the arms. Keep your elbows tucked in as you push back up through your hands.

> *Joanna's top tip:* This may look easy, but positioning the cushion means you can't cheat—check you keep your neck long and avoid hunching your ears down by your shoulders as you perform this exercise.

COOLING DOWN

Don't forget to cool down after each Total Body Solution workout. For ease, you can repeat your warm-up in reverse, decreasing the size of your movements and then finishing off with the stretches below. Each stretch position is multi-functional, lengthening and stretching more than one body part. Hold each stretch position for 10–30 seconds.

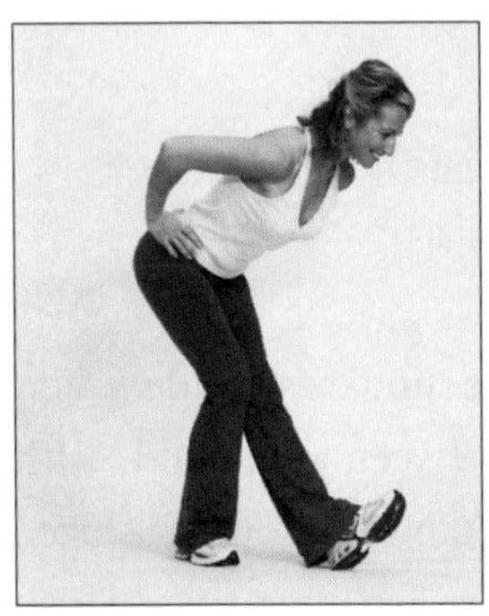

Exercise: Standing leg stretch

Stretches: Calves and hamstrings

Stand with good posture. Extend one leg in front of you, flexing the foot at the ankle. Bend your back knee and flex forward from the hips, contracting your abdominals as you extend forward. Lift up from the hips, checking they are level. Imagine you are balancing two glasses of water on each side of your lower back to help you. To progress the stretch, lift your leg and rest it on a bench, low step, or chair.

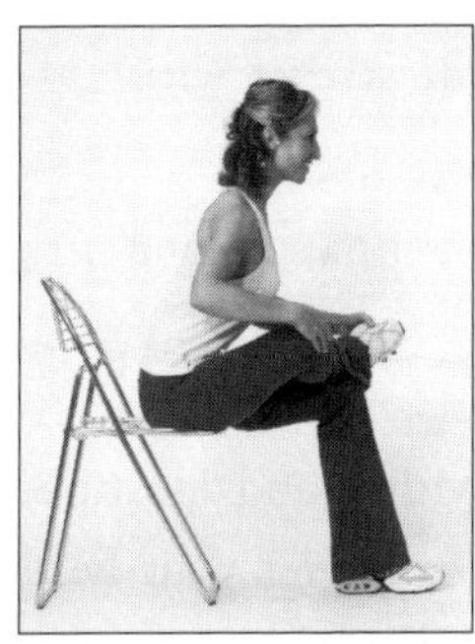

Exercise: Seated buttock stretch

Stretches: Buttocks and chest

Sit on a chair with good posture. Cross one ankle and rest it on the other knee. Lean forward from the hips, extending tall through your spine, until you feel a stetch on your buttocks and outer hip. Draw your shoulders back to open and stretch your chest. To progress the stretch you can bring your weight onto your elbows; you should feel a deep stretch on the buttock of the crossed leg and across your chest.

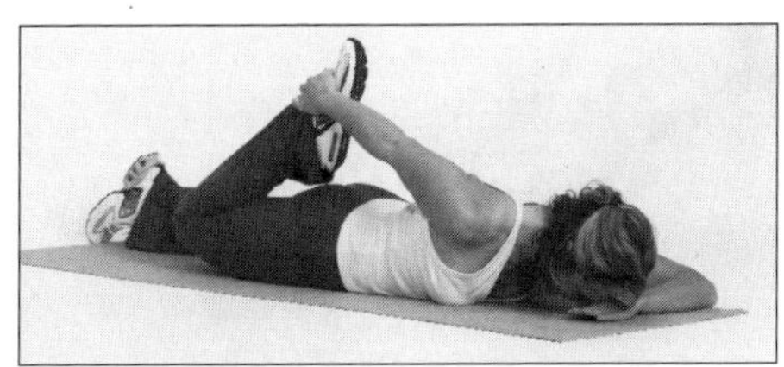

Exercise: Lying quad stretch

Stretches: Front thigh and hip flexor

Lie face-down on the floor. Contract your abdominals to support your spine. Lift one leg into your butt and reach back with the same hand as the lifted leg to hold on to the ankle or shoelaces. Keep your knees together and press your hips into the floor to increase the stretch.

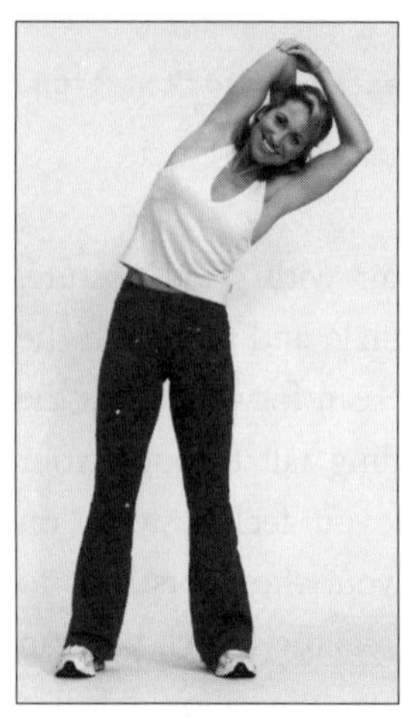

Exercise: Side stretch with triceps

Stretches: Waist muscles and back of arms.

Standing with good posture, extend one arm over your head and drop the hand between your shoulder blades. Support it with the other hand as you lean away from the elevated arm.

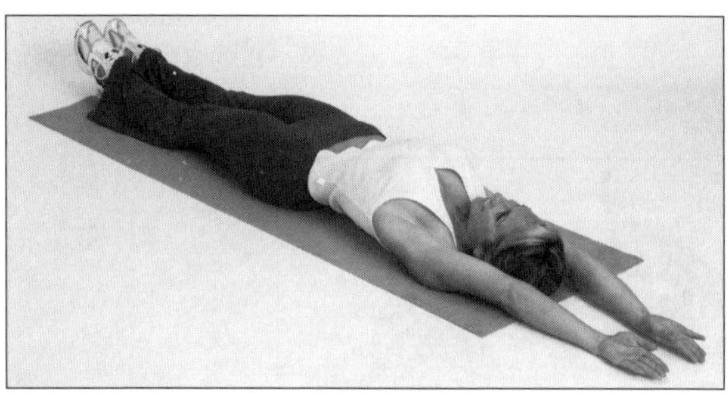

Exercise: Lying full-body stretch

Stretches: Abdominals, thighs and shoulders

Lie on the floor face-up. Extend your arms above your head. Gently stretch and lengthen through your whole body from your fingertips to toes. Your lower back may come gently off the floor. Breathe gently and hold for up to 30 seconds. Slowly bring your arms down by your side.

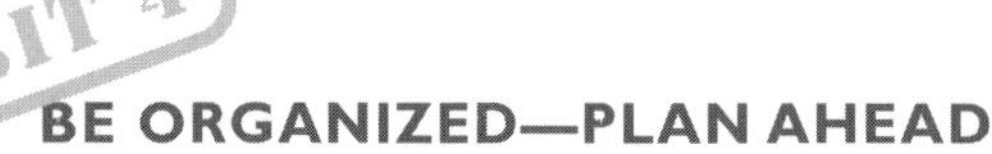

BE ORGANIZED—PLAN AHEAD

This strategy is all about being prepared. Prior preparation prevents poor performance—so the saying goes, and there is a lot of truth to it. If, for example, you had decided to start the *Get a Grip* plan and only read the instructions on Monday morning, you may well have decided not to bother, as you didn't have the right foods in the house, hadn't time to fit in a walk, hadn't prepared any soup, and so on. You'd be far more likely to get off on the right foot if you had read the information through a few days before and got prepared. The same goes for exercise. A study on marathon runners in Japan found that those who dropped out during the race were those who had prepared least in training!

Developing the "being prepared" habit focuses on two areas: being prepared with your food and exercise, and being prepared to deal with temptation.

PUTTING PLANNING INTO PRACTICE

PLAN YOUR MEALS

No one wants to come in from a busy day and spend hours in the kitchen. Having an idea of what you are going to cook is important in making sure you have the necessary ingredients, and also being pre-warned of the time needed for marinading, chopping, and so on. For those days when time really is at a premium, check out our *On Your Plate in 15 minutes* recipes on page 225 for some really fast, easy, and nutritious Starch Curfew supper ideas.

SHOPPING

If you are the sort of person who rushes to the store on the way home to grab something for dinner, you may need to change your habits a little in order to achieve and maintain your weight-loss goals. Why? Well, you're more likely to find yourself in the local fast-food place if you've had a tiring day than buying things to cook if you never had a plan of what you were going to eat. Secondly, many late-opening stores have a poor selection of fresh vegetables and fruits. Writing a shopping list is essential—it will insure you have what you need for the week ahead and it will also stop you wandering aimlessly up the aisles and being tempted by unhealthy food choices. Your shopping cart should contain 40 percent fruit and vegetables, but these don't all need to be fresh—frozen, canned, and dried count, too. OK, you may need fresh vegetables for your salads, but think about frozen bags of fruit for smoothies, canned vegetables for adding to soups and stews, and frozen vegetables as accompaniments to your Starch Curfew suppers.

I'm a busy mom with a part-time job, and feeding Jamie and Charlotte was always a rush—it just seemed so much easier to give them franks and beans and have supper with them. I thought because I was having oven fries instead of deep-frying them, I was doing myself a real favor! I never thought I had the time to shop and cook healthily. Now I buy bags of pre-cut fresh and frozen vegetables, cooked chicken pieces and throw them all together in a stir-fry—it can be on the table in 10 minutes. I've even got into the habit of cooking a bit of extra rice to use the following day for my lunch—I add it to my soups or make a salad and take it to work. I've saved time and money and kept my weight off for 12 months—a total of 28 pounds. **Emmaline, 28**

DELIVER ME FROM TEMPTATION!

Being prepared is not just about having the right foods on hand to help you select better choices. It is also about understanding how your body responds to temptation and the challenges you will come across. It's actually far easier to "beat" temptation if you are expecting it. Think about this: when is your willpower strongest to avoid temptation? Chances are, it will be at the start of the day—you may not necessarily be a morning person, but most people tend to find it easier to make healthier decisions in the morning. "I'll opt for cereal and fruit for breakfast, rather than a Danish pastry on the way to work" for example. As the day progresses and your energy levels start to flag, your willpower may start to dwindle, too, to the point that you can no longer resist the call of the candy machine by 4 p.m. If this is particularly pertinent to you, you may find the *Damage Limitation* section particularly helpful.

The brain is one of the most energy-demanding parts

of the body. It requires a constant flow of energy in the form of blood sugar. When our blood sugar drops too low, our ability to concentrate is directly affected and our willpower is greatly challenged. Maintaining stable blood sugar levels can help you sustain willpower. To achieve this, you need do three things:

1. Operate the Starch Curfew (see page 108)
2. Boost your intake of slow-releasing carbohydrates (see page 110)
3. Focus on your food ratios, especially at lunchtime (see number 8 page 157)
4. Keep well hydrated (see page 144)

TAKING ON TEMPTATION

CREATE DISTANCE

If you can't resist the urge to dig into the cookie jar, then you need to create some distance between yourself and the jar. By distance, I mean not just putting the jar out of sight but creating a "time distance" as well, to give you a little more time to get your willpower to kick in. Rather than telling yourself "No, I can't have a cookie," say to yourself "If I still really want one by the time I have taken those clothes upstairs and got the washing out of the machine, then I'll reconsider." By then, you may have summoned enough willpower to forgo the cookie jar or, even better, you may have forgotten about it altogether!

I knew I had a problem with the cookie jar, so after trying many tricks to deny myself, I decided to put the jar in the closet with the ironing board and all the ironing. I knew I would have to face the task of doing the ironing every time I went to the closet for a cookie. The strategy worked! Some days I don't even open the closet door as I don't want to look at the ironing and on other days I open the door intending to have a cookie and my willpower kicks in—instead of digging into the cookies I plow into my husband's shirts! On other days I set myself a target of ironing five shirts, taking them up and down the stairs and then allowing myself a cookie. By the time I get that done—I often find the urge has gone. **Penny, 48**

RATE YOUR HUNGER

When hunger appears to strike, ask yourself if you are *really* hungry, or if you are actually bored, or thirsty, or just plain putting off a job you don't really want to do. If you can genuinely say you are hungry, then fine—have something to eat, prepare it and sit down to eat it. This is a far healthier strategy than simply popping food in your mouth and then being racked with guilt 20 minutes later when you realize you didn't really want it.

If, when you do start to eat, you find yourself overeating and unable to stop, try "rating your hunger". This is a really clever little trick. Before you eat, rate how hungry you are: 0 means you are famished while 5 means you are absolutely stuffed. Choose which number most closely represents how you feel. Studies have shown individuals who wait until their hunger rating is 0 before they eat actually take in more calories and are more likely to eat to a hunger rating of 5 (overeat) than individuals who sit down to eat when their hunger rating is 2.

So try to eat when you have a hunger rating of 2, but stop when you have a hunger rating of 4. As my grandfather used to say to my mom, you should always leave the table feeling you could eat just a little bit more.

LEARN TO SELF-TALK

This strategy is all about being prepared to give yourself a good talking to! When that little voice tries to lure you away from your good intentions, you need to be able to rationalize temptation and muster up willpower. For example, you set the alarm 10 minutes early, intending to go for a 10-minute power walk before you shower and go to work. But the alarm goes off and you think—I'll have the extra 10 minutes in bed and walk later. This is where developing self-talk is important. The following example illustrates how you can develop self-talk for yourself:

The alarm goes off …

You: I think I'll exercise later and have the extra snooze.

Self-talk: No, get up now and do it now—you know your day will get busy later on.

You: But I'm tired! I need the extra sleep.

Self-talk: An extra 10 minutes will not get rid of your

tiredness, and besides, getting active is a great way to energize yourself.

You: But I'll do it later, after work.

Self-talk: You know that last time you did that, your day got too busy and your willpower was low, so you never did it. You might as well get up and do it now!

This is a simple scenario, but developing self-talk through rationalization will help you be prepared and overcome the temptation to duck out of your good intentions.

HABIT 5
DRINK MORE WATER

Almost two-thirds of our body weight consists of it, every single cell is bathed in it, and every single process in our bodies requires its presence. What is it? Water. And yet this vital nutrient is the one we most often overlook. If you rarely drink water, and instead quench thirst with tea, coffee or colas, you are probably in a constant state of dehydration. Not only does this prevent your body functioning optimally, it can also hamper your weight-loss efforts, as fat can only be broken down in the presence of water. Study findings estimate that 30–40 percent of us are mildly to moderately dehydrated. Research suggests we need 1ml of fluid per calorie of energy we consume. So if your average daily intake is 1600 calories, you need a minimum of 1.6 litres (7 cups) of water. While a balanced diet containing lots of fruit and vegetables can provide a proportion of this fluid, we should balance these sources with drinking water itself.

Adequate water consumption is even more important if you are a regular caffeine or alcohol drinker, as these substances both have a diuretic effect (meaning they cause your body to *lose* water). A study found that drinking six cups of coffee a day increased urinary excretion by 3⅓ cups! A good rule of thumb is to consume one glass of water for every cup of caffeinated or alcoholic drink and to keep these to a minimum.

You may well have found that, initially, the water you drank during the 14-day plan had you in and out of the bathroom, but as your body becomes accustomed to consuming 9 cups of water a day, this will wear off. Hopefully, you're now significantly more active than you were before you started the plan—this too will have a bearing on how much water you need. If you are regularly active it is likely that you will need more than 9 cups of water a day to stay properly hydrated—we lose 2¼-4½ cups of fluid per hour of exercise. A level of just 2 percent dehydration will undermine your body's ability to perform exercise. To offset this loss, aim to drink 1 cup every 15 minutes during a workout. Don't wait until you are thirsty—thirst is the body's last response to dehydration. Additionally, your brain can interpret thirst signals as hunger, and this can cause unhealthy snacking. Your brain may be telling you to drink more water, but if you have got out of the habit, your brain will misinterpret this message as a need to eat more.

As you re-educate your thirst mechanism, you'll find it easier to understand what your body needs to keep your energy levels up.

One way of revealing how much water your body has lost during exercise is to weigh yourself before and after a vigorous exercise session. And yes, any change in your body weight is *solely* due to loss of fluid, as changes in fat and muscle composition don't come until later.

PUTTING THE WATER HABIT INTO PRACTICE

Much of the battle with adopting this strategy is simply getting used to it. It's not about denying yourself something or having to take time out to do something—it's simply about getting into the habit of remembering to drink it. Don't make the mistake of trying to drink a day's water allocation all at once. Not only is this not an effective way for you to maintain hydration, it will also make you feel bloated and uncomfortable, especially if you're about to do some exercise. Have a bottle of water on your desk at work, by the telephone at home, and always carry a bottle in your bag.

When I first started the plan I couldn't imagine how I was ever going to be able to drink all that water. I felt like all I was doing was drinking water or going to the bathroom! I have always drunk lots of tea and coffee but I found that restricting my intake to 2 (or sometimes 3) cups a day improved my energy levels and mood. I now carry a small bottle of water in my bag, always drink water with my meals and take a glass to bed with me every night. For someone who never touched the stuff a few weeks ago, that's pretty good going! **Joan, 63**

Devise a "trigger" so that every time you do a particular thing (such as go to the bathroom, make a phone call or put the cat out) you automatically drink a glass of water. If you're at work, aim to drink a glass for every hour that you are there—then you should be able to achieve the minimum 8 glasses a day.

WHICH WATER?

Any water is better than no water, regardless of whether it comes from a faucet, a filter jug, or a bottle. Carbonated water is not absorbed by the body tissues as quickly as still water, although it's fine to include some in your daily quota if you enjoy the taste. Experts also believe that water is best absorbed when drunk at room temperature rather than straight from the fridge. Research shows that the number-one reason people fail to drink enough water is the taste—or lack of taste. Add a squeeze of lime or lemon, or infuse a slice of fresh ginger if you think water tastes too dull on its own. And drinking water is important for children, too! Studies have shown that orange and grape flavors can be the most effective for stimulating a child to drink.

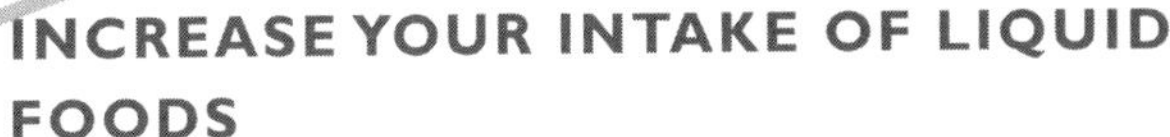

INCREASE YOUR INTAKE OF LIQUID FOODS

As you may have noticed, the 14-day plan included a high proportion of liquid-based foods, such as soups, juices, and smoothies, as well as water-based vegetables and fruit. This is a strategy well worth maintaining. Not only does it insure you consume a large variety and volume of vitamin-packed fruits and vegetables, it can also assist your weight-loss efforts.

TAKE YOUR FILL

You may well have found that the daily soup before your evening meal helped you feel full—especially in the absence of starchy accompaniments to your dinner. Well, if so, it's no surprise, as research from Penn State University found that foods with a high water content help stave off hunger. In the study, women who were served a soup prior to their meal ate fewer calories than those who were served a drier appetizer along with a glass of water.

The same team of researchers found that basing meals on water-packed foods enabled dieters to stick to a diet plan without feeling deprived or feeling that they had had to cut portion sizes dramatically. It makes sense: picture a sandwich filled with ham and a scrape of mustard. Now picture a sandwich containing a slice of ham and water-packed vegetables such as arugula leaves, tomato, onion, and beetroot. It's easy to imagine which would leave you feeling more satisfied, not just physically but mentally, too.

We've already talked about the importance of water consumption as part of a healthy lifestyle, but water shouldn't replace liquid-based foods as a weight-loss strategy—the Penn State researchers found that drinking water with meals wasn't effective in reducing calorie intake.

Oh, and a word of warning—liquid-based foods doesn't mean liquid lunches! A study in the *American Journal of Clinical Nutrition* found that just a single pre-lunch wine or beer resulted in less post-meal satiety and increased calorie intake over the next 24 hours.

PUTTING THE LIQUID FOODS STRATEGY INTO PRACTICE

First and foremost, don't drop the juices and soups from your daily diet—even if you're not hungry—and make sure you include fruits and vegetables from the suggested lists to accompany your meals. The varieties selected are particularly high in water, so they'll make you feel fuller than other types.

The mid-morning juice and pre-dinner soup definitely helped me to stick with the plan. Just as hunger began to strike, I'd remember to have my juice and then I'd feel able to carry on until lunchtime. The soup insures you don't feel deprived at dinnertime and, for me, that was really important as I was wondering how I would ever cope with potato- or rice-free meals! **Sam, 33**

If you're pushed for time, prepare the fruit or vegetables you need for the juices in the morning so you can just throw them in the juicer or blender when you want them. Or fall back on a store-bought option. When you make a soup, make a lot and freeze what you don't need for the next few days. For variety, make a couple of different recipes and freeze them in small boxes so that you don't have to have the same one every night. Check out the recipe section in the appendices for more tasty, filling soup and smoothie recipes.

Another easy way to include more liquid-based foods in your daily diet is by checking out the incredibly simple liquid-based meal options in the table overleaf. These can work as starch curfew soups and stews or filling lunches, depending on when you choose to eat them. If it's for lunch, add half a cup of cooked pasta or brown rice to your soup as it cooks, 2 chopped boiled potatoes, or 2 tablespoons of barley. Alternatively, serve with a whole-wheat brown roll. They are all quick to make, nutritious, and versatile. Enjoy!

QUICK AND EASY LIQUID MEALS

This is so simple—all you do is:

1. Take a soup base
2. Add a protein option
3. Chuck in a vegetable option, eat and enjoy!

Follow the ideas or make up your own quick and easy liquid meals.

Soup base	Protein option	Vegetable option	What you do
Tomato and Basil	Cottage cheese	Chopped tomatoes and fresh basil	Heat the soup, add the chopped tomatoes and heat through. Pour into a bowl, top with the cottage cheese and sprinkle with the fresh basil.
Carrot and Cilantro	Canned chickpeas	Leeks, carrots, and onions	In a non-stick pan, soften the chopped onion, carrot, and leeks. When soft, add the soup and drained chickpeas. Heat thoroughly and serve. Feeling fancy? Garnish with a tablespoon of yogurt and sprinkle of cumin.
Chilled cucumber	Canned salmon	Cucumber and broccoli	Heat the soup, add the chopped cucumber and broccoli and cook until the vegetables are *al dente*. Add the drained salmon and heat through. Feeling fancy? Serve with chopped cucumber on top with a drizzle of Thai sweet chili sauce.

Soup base	Protein option	Vegetable option	What you do
Chicken and corn	Chicken breast	Snowpeas, canned or fresh corn	In a non-stick pan, soften the snowpeas and corn over a moderate heat. Add the chicken breast and stir. Heat thoroughly and serve. Add a little soy sauce to the snowpeas and chicken while heating for a bit of a Chinese flavor.
Tomato, red pepper, and lime	Mixed seafood (mussels, shrimp, calamari, cockles)	Onion and red pepper	In a non-stick pan, soften the chopped onion and red pepper over a moderate heat. Stir in a tablespoon of Thai sweet chili sauce. Add the seafood and heat thoroughly. Stir in the soup and heat through.
Tomato	Canned tuna	Watercress and cucumber	Chop the watercress and steam with the cucumber in a little water. Add the soup and drained tuna and heat thoroughly. Serve with a dollop of natural yogurt.

Soup base	Protein option	Vegetable option	What you do
Mushroom	Cold roast lean beef	Mushrooms—different types work particularly well	In a non-stick pan, soften the mushrooms. Add the chopped meat and the soup and heat through. Serve with chopped raw mushrooms, or, for extra zing, you can sauté the mushrooms in a little garlic and hot grainy mustard.
Gazpacho	Hard-boiled egg	Chopped red onion, red and yellow pepper, and cucumber	Pour the soup into a bowl, garnish with the chopped vegetables and top with the chopped boiled egg.

With the exception of the Gazpacho, remember to heat all the soups thoroughly before serving. Do not boil soups excessively, however, as this can damage the flavor.

HABIT 7
TIME YOUR EXERCISE TO SUIT YOU

In *Get a Grip*, we aimed to get you active as early in the day as possible. Not only does getting off on the right foot help you stick with the plan all day, evidence shows that people who exercise in the morning are more likely to stick with a long-term program. It makes sense, as first thing, there are fewer obstacles to get between you and your workout. We also spread bouts of activity throughout the day, as these are often easier to fit in than one extended exercise session.

If, after the two-week plan, you still find "early bird" exercise a pain, worry not! Research on performance and time of day suggests that we can work *harder* without perceiving it to be so in the late afternoon to early evening. A study from the University of North Texas found that volunteers were able to work 26 percent harder in the afternoon than in the morning, which perhaps helps suggest why most Olympic records have been set in the late afternoon and early evening. Other research shows that our body's aerobic system responds to exercise more quickly in the afternoon compared to the morning. As far as how often you exercise during the day goes, some research suggests that the effect on metabolism of repeated bouts of exercise is greater than when you restrict physical activity to just one daily slot. If you are continuing to exercise in small bouts, aim to keep them to 15–20 minutes. A study found that 5–10 minute bouts, while having a beneficial effect on metabolism, did not have such a strong impact on blood lipids (fats). The overall message is to do what works for you. If your body tells you that exercise is easier and more enjoyable in the evening, then plan your day to include a later workout. If you'd rather grab 10 minutes every few hours than put aside a whole hour, fine. Fit in exercise where you can. The fact that you're doing it is far more important than time of day.

PUTTING SUITABLE TIMING INTO PRACTICE

Experiment with exercise at different times of day. You may surprise yourself by finding you love the peace and quiet of the early morning for a power walk or enjoy winding down with a late evening yoga class. Contrary to popular belief, light exercise before bedtime doesn't keep you awake—in fact, one study found that it helped subjects get off to the land of Nod more quickly *and* enhanced the quality of their sleep.

Listen to your body—if you need to go more gently in the morning (research shows that it takes us longer to get going in the morning as we age) then do so. Muscles and joints are at their stiffest early on, too, so make sure you're thoroughly warmed up before stretching. As far as muscles go, experts say that strength peaks in the afternoon to early evening. Why not try the Total Body Solution workout (page 120) in this time slot and see if it feels easier?

Do what you can, when you can—it may end up being all you do if the trials and tribulations of the day get in the way. If you don't seize an exercise opportunity when you can, you may miss out altogether. While it is often recommended that you try to spread your exercise sessions throughout the week, it won't make much difference in physical terms. Studies do show, however, that people tend to feel they've achieved more when they are able to spread exercise evenly throughout the week.

Although I am not what you'd call a morning person, I made the effort to get up and do the pre-breakfast walk and abdominal exercises. This helped me to remain positive throughout the 14 days as if work got really busy and stressful and prevented me from doing any more walking, I knew that I'd at least done something. **Sam, 33**

HABIT 8

FIGURE OUT YOUR FOODS

It's fairly obvious that in order to lose weight and body fat, you need to use more calories than you are consuming. This needs to be achieved through a combination of sensible nutrition and physical exercise. To reduce body fat you need to create a deficit of 3500 calories a week. This figure can appear alarming, but don't panic! The secret to effective weight and body-fat loss is to make sure that the calorie burn is achieved slowly and consistently. Spreading the 3500 calories over seven days means you are aiming for a decrease of 500 calories each day. If you split these 500 calories between physical activity, structured exercise and nutritional habit building, it becomes a lot more manageable. You do *not* need to put your life on hold to reach your healthy weight and body-fat goals.

GETTING THE BALANCE RIGHT

Many people experience changes in their energy levels when they start a "diet". Feelings of tiredness can relate to the fact that the body is having to survive on fewer calories than it is used to. Nutritional Habit Building is not about getting you to continually survive on fewer and fewer calories, but about learning to apply techniques that help you match your energy intake with the amount of energy you need. In this section, I'll explain how you can figure out your foods in relation to the different properties and calorie values of the main nutrient groups—and why you need the right balance of all three. If you look back at *Get a Grip*, you'll see many of the volunteers commented on how much more energy they had. This in part relates to the fact that they were eating the right nutrients in the right ratios at the right time.

WHERE DOES ENERGY COME FROM?

The main food groups—proteins, fats, and carbohydrates—provide the body with energy. The body uses this energy to carry out its everyday activities, from going to pick up the kids from school, completing structured exercise, and even digesting your food. Energy is measured in calories, but not all foods give the same amount of energy. You'll see from the table below that one gram of fat provides nearly twice the amount of energy as one gram of protein. (Alcohol also provides the body with energy—7 cals per gram—but it is not a nutrient as it is not necessary for life.)

Nutrient	**Energy per gram** Cals
Carbohydrate	4
Fat	9
Protein	4

The amount of calories you are eating is important, but it is not the whole story when it comes to sustaining a healthy diet—different foods, and combinations of foods, affect the rate at which your body receives energy and even affect the brain differently. This is a fascinating area, and once you have learned to balance your food intake, you will really notice a huge difference in your ability to concentrate and maintain motivation.

You learned about the Glycemic Index in section two, so you know that some foods produce a sharp rise in blood sugar and a subsequent dip in energy, often accompanied by cravings for more starchy foods. But did you know that many starch-rich foods such as bread, pasta, rice, and potatoes increase the amount of serotonin your body produces? This brain transmitter has a "calming" effect, and can cause feelings of lethargy. If you have ever experienced that post-lunch slump—a feeling of wanting to put your head down on your desk or eat a chunk of chocolate to give you "energy" to get through the afternoon (even though you have just had your lunch!)—you may be getting your food ratios wrong.

Starch-based foods do provide us with an important energy source, but the trick is to get the balance right, and this is where food ratios come in.

It is a really simple concept that involves eating an equal amount of protein with your starch. This slows down the release of blood sugar, dampens the effect of serotonin and helps maintain your energy levels.

Ideally, your lunchtime meal should include an equal amount of protein and starch—that means a ratio of one to one. You don't need to weigh things out to achieve this —you can simply estimate it by what the foods look like. Take a ham sandwich as an example. The sandwich has two slices of bread (the starch) and a slice of ham (protein);

the ratio is therefore two to one. To get a better ratio, ditch the top slice of bread and add a slice more ham so it looks about the same quantity as the slice of bread. Now add a side salad or pile on a bag of salad with chopped tomatoes and peppers and you have got yourself a perfect one-to-one food ratio lunch. The great thing about food ratios is that it works for everyone: the whole family can benefit even if they do not want to lose weight—all you have to do is give them an equal amount of starch and protein at lunch.

Starch isn't the only energy-influencing nutrient. Protein-rich foods such as chicken, tofu, fish, lean red meat, and legumes stimulate the release of dopamine in the brain, which increases our ability to concentrate and focus. Make sure you get sufficient protein in your diet, whether it is from meat and fish sources or legumes and vegetables. It is important for everyone to have a varied diet of fruit and vegetables, as eating too much protein decreases the body's ability to absorb vitamin C and vitamin B. Absorption of these two vitamins is especially suppressed if you suffer from stress. In these situations, the body actually produces more homocysteine, a compound that has been implicated in an increased risk of heart disease. Eating a diet rich in fruit and vegetables will help you increase your intake of vitamins C and B and readdress the balance—another reason why the Starch Curfew is beneficial to your health!

FIGURING OUT FATS

As you can see from the table above, the fat in our food is the most concentrated source of energy (calories). But this is not to say we should be cutting out all fat in the diet. Nearly all of us need to decrease our fat intake, but it is not a case of having no fat. Some fat is important for normal health—it protects organs like the liver and kidneys, it plays a role in enabling and sustaining pregnancy, and it helps keep us warm. Some vitamins—A, D, E, and K—are "fat-soluble", meaning that fat must be present in order for them to be used by the body. Some foods contain essential fats, which our bodies cannot make themselves. In addition, research has shown an association between depression and very low-fat diets.

So how much is enough? Ideally, total fat intake should provide no more than 30 percent of the total calories in our diet. This means that if your calorie intake falls within the recommended female daily requirements of 1900–2100 calories per day, then you should be consuming *no more than* 63–72 grams of fat per day. For a male, the recommended daily requirements are 2100–2500 calories per day, allowing 70–83 grams of fat per day. A study of 2200 British adults found that the average intake of fat for women was 74 grams, and for men, 102 grams per day. Check out the table below to see how replacing a fattening favorite with a healthy alternative a few times a week can make a difference to your weight ...

Fattening Favorite	Tasty Alternative	Calories saved if you swop your fattening fave for your tasty alternative twice a week	Over the course of a year, you'll save yourself ... (remember, 3500 calories = 1lb of fat!)	Potential weight loss over 1 year
Chunk of cheese (1oz) 115 cals	Low-fat cheese 75 cals	80 cals	4160 cals	1.2lb
1 chocolate cookie 85 cals	1 cracker 55 cals	60 cals	3120 cals	0.9lb
Large handful of tortilla chips 245 cals	Large handful of plain popcorn 165 cals	160 cals	8320 cals	2.4lb
Rich and creamy rice pudding (½ can) 190 cals	Canned peaches with 4oz pot of fruit yogurt 90 cals	200 cals	10,400 cals	3lb
1 shrimp and egg deep-filled sandwich 570 cals	Low-fat shrimp, lemon and chili mayo sandwich, 265 cals	710 cals	36,920 cals	10.5lb
½ pot taramasalata 400 cals	½ pot reduced-fat hummus 210 cals	380 cals	19,760 cals	5.6lb

For weight-management purposes, I recommend a daily fat intake of 30–40 grams. However, all fats are not created equal and in your efforts to reduce fat intake it is best to focus on specific types of fat. These include saturated and trans fat sources. Other types of fats, such as essential fatty acids found in oily fish, should be maintained or even increased. For health purposes, fat intake should never fall below 10 grams a day.

FIGURE OUT YOUR FATS

Check out the table opposite to learn more about the different types of fat in our diet and which ones to approach with caution.

Note: The polyunsaturated essential fatty acids—omega-6 and omega-3—are considered "essential" because our bodies are unable to manufacture them. They must therefore be obtained from our diet.

ALWAYS READ THE LABEL

Food labels can be very misleading. For example, peanut butter labels may read "cholesterol free"—this is true, but the peanut butter never had cholesterol in it in the first place! And cholesterol free does *not* mean fat free. Some cereal manufacturers claim "no added fat" on granola or wholesome cereal products, yet the natural grains have been processed with coconut or palm oils, which are high in saturated fat. One food may be described on the label as "low fat" but in actual fact this may be a relative

Fat Type	Typical Sources	Health Effect	Recommendations
Saturated Fat	Meat, dairy products and some tropical oils including palm oil and cocoa butter	Increases cholestrol levels. Increases risk of heart disease and certain cancers	The less the better. No more than 10% of total calories. (In a 1000-cal diet that would be 10g—equivalent to 2 tsps!)
Trans Fatty Acids—mostly man-made molecules produced during hydrogenation of vegetable oil, a process used in the manufacture of various foodstuffs including margarine	Margarine, shortening, fried foods, breads, crackers, snack foods, spreads, processed/prepared foods	Has a negative effect on cholesterol—decreases the HDL (good) and increases the LDL (bad). May increase risk of heart disease and breast cancer	The less the better, minimize consumption. Avoid products that use the words "hydrogenated" or "partially hydrogenated" on the label
Monounsaturated Fatty Acids	Olive, canola, almond, cashew, hazelnut, macadamia, pecan and peanut oils	Has a beneficial effect on cholesterol levels. Lowers LDL and maintains HDL	Olive oil and canola oil are the best choices. Should make up 12% of total calories

Fat Type	Typical Sources	Health Effect	Recommendations
POLYUNSATURATED FATS			
Omega-6 Essential Fatty Acids	Corn, safflower, sesame, soybean, sunflower oils, nuts and wheatgerm	Consuming too many of these vegetable oils can alter the delicate balance of omega-6 and omega-3 fats	Limit consumption of these vegetable oils—should make up no more than 10% of total calories. Avoid heating these delicate oils—instead use olive oil or canola oil for cooking
Omega-3 Essential Fatty Acids	Cold-water fish (salmon, mackerel, herring, halibut, tuna and sardines). Flaxseed, hempseed, walnuts and their oils, soybean oils, green leafy vegetables	Inhibits blood clots, reduces risk of heart disease, increases immune function	Increase consumption to 3–6g daily. (Have oily fish 3 times a week or 1 tsp freshly ground flaxseed daily)

term comparing what is essentially a high-fat food to the even higher fat standard product. Mayonnaise is a classic example of this—even the "low fat" version can hardly be described as low in calories.

The information on food labels can help you compare the types and amount of fat in specific foods.

Here are some quick guidelines to look for:

1. Look at total fat intake and not just saturated fat. Any fat, healthy or not, provides 9 calories per gram.
2. Just because it says "low fat" on the front does not necessarily mean it is a low-fat food. An apple is a naturally low-fat food while "low-fat" mayo is not!
3. Avoid trans fats by looking for the term "hydrogenated". The higher up the list you see this term, the more hydrogenated unhealthy fats are in the food.
4. It may say "reduced fat" on the label but do check out the total calories—the extra flavor may be added through the use of extra sugars and processed flavorings.

HABIT 9

EXERCISE PORTION CONTROL

Few people know what a "standard" portion looks like. In experiments in which people are asked to prepare a standard-sized meal, the vast majority cook up portions

2–3 times the size recommended by government health guidelines. It's not really surprising—eat out at a restaurant or get take-out and you'll frequently be served a meal big enough for two or three people. A coffee shop "tall" coffee can contain three times the amount of caffeine of a standard cup. A study in the *American Journal of Public Health* recently found that in the States, portion sizes are 2–5 times bigger than they were 30 years ago—and judging from the burgeoning problem with obesity, the people who are eating them are, too! The amount you eat is important, regardless of what the food is. Take white bread, for example—a basic foodstuff in most people's kitchen containing no fat. Yet if you eat enough of it, you'll gain weight. The same goes for apples, chicken breasts, oatmeal—you name it. The fact is we have to exercise portion control in order to achieve weight control.

Since completing the 14-day plan, you probably have a far better idea of portion sizes. To help you maintain a visual picture of what a standard portion of a particular food looks like—so that you don't get led astray by gigantic restaurant or take-out portions—we've included a reference list of food portions sized by everyday household objects.

PORTION SIZES IN THE REAL WORLD

Cheese—a matchbox-sized piece (30g/1oz) equals one serving

Rice—your fist equates to about a cup, a standard portion of rice should be ½ cup (uncooked)
Pasta—a helping the size of your computer mouse when uncooked
Fish—a piece the size of a woman's palm (85g/3oz) equals one serving
Meat or poultry—a piece the size of a credit card, about 2.5cm/½ inch thick (85g/3oz) equals one serving
1 bagel—the size of a compact disc
1 slice of pizza—should be no bigger than a standard white business envelope

When I started the plan and prepared some of the recipes included, I was amazed at how small the portions appeared to be. It would say "serves 4" when I'd think there was just about enough for two! Yet, once supplemented with a juicy salad or some tasty vegetables I found the meals recommended to be perfectly satisfying. I realized then how big the helpings I'd been eating before were. **Sam, 33**

PUTTING PORTION CONTROL INTO PRACTICE

- Get into the habit of weighing foods to see how much constitutes a single serving. You won't need to do it forever, as you'll soon be familiar enough with the amounts to simply estimate them.
- When you've prepared and served your recommended helping size of a particular meal, put the remainder away immediately.

If you leave the bowl on the table or the bread on the breadboard you'll be tempted to have a little bit extra.

- Serve your meal on a smaller plate so that it fills it up. No matter how appetizing it smells, a small meal on a vast white plate isn't the most appealing prospect.

HABIT 10

EAT PLENTY OF FIBER

The high intake of fruit and vegetables in the *Get a Grip* plan insured that your intake of fiber was high. Studies show that foods rich in fiber tend to be more bulky and less calorie-dense than low-fiber foods. They take longer to chew and they slow the rate of digestion (and therefore blood sugar release) down, enabling you to feel fuller for longer. The result? You are less likely to overeat. Research from Penn State University in the United States found that fiber was one of the key secrets in feeling satiated while reducing calorie intake. There are other benefits to be gained, too. In a study of 139 people, those who started eating cereal packed with 6–12g of fiber daily reported feeling more energetic than those who began the day with a low-fiber cereal. Asked to rate their energy levels, the high-fiber crowd gave themselves scores 10 percent higher than the low-fiber-eating group. They also reported feeling better and thinking more clearly.

Why? Most likely, at least in part, by alleviating that

common little problem that no one likes to talk about: constipation. Studies report that individuals who switch to high-fiber diets feel more energetic because they feel lighter and more comfortable. The average diet contains around 13g of fiber or less a day. This has been associated with stool weights of less than 100g a day, which, in turn, have been linked to a raised risk of bowel disease. Eating more fiber can also help lower the risk of diabetes, heart disease, and possibly cancer, and can help control your weight. In addition, soluble fiber, such as that found in oatmeal and legumes, is thought to have a beneficial effect on cholesterol levels.

HOW MUCH FIBER DO I NEED?

You should be getting 18–32g a day. Increasing your fiber intake to 18g a day translates into a 25 percent increase in stool weight. It might not sound like a very attractive prospect, but it will make you feel healthier and more energetic. You may find it takes your system a few days to adjust to a higher fiber intake, but stay with it. In the study mentioned above, the high-fiber group did experience more abdominal bloating at first, but this eased during the second week.

PUTTING FIBER ON THE MENU

Getting more fiber in your diet doesn't mean eating bowlfuls of bran and munching on celery sticks all day long. You can increase fiber intake by making a few small changes to your shopping and eating habits. Here are a few ideas:

- Opt for whole-wheat flour instead of white flour in baking and choose whole-wheat bread instead of white, most of the time.
- Use whole-wheat varieties of rice and pasta. Whole-wheat pasta has 3.5 grams of fiber per 100g compared to just 1.2 grams in white pasta.
- Serve every meal with a variety of vegetables or salad—scrape rather than peel, or leave skins intact to retain the maximum amount of fiber.
- Ensure you eat at least 3 pieces of fruit a day—oranges are particularly high in fiber, as are berry fruits such as raspberries, and dried fruits and golden raisins pack a fiber punch in a concentrated form.

Breakfast is an ideal opportunity to add more fiber to your diet. A single bowl of high-fiber cereal can narrow the deficit.

If you like …	**Switch to …**	**Your Fiber Boost …**
Crunchy Nut cornflakes 0.9g	Bran Flakes 4.2g	3.3g
Special K 0.8g	Fruit & Fibre 2.7g	1.9g
Rice Krispies 0.5g	Shredded Wheat Spoon Size 3.4g	2.9g

Hopefully, you have started to build some of these habits already. Over the next few weeks and months, try to add in one more strategy to your weight-loss efforts until they all become regular practice. Don't worry if some take longer to get the hang of than others, and don't beat yourself up if you go off track every now and then. Accept that accidents do occur, and simply get back to your new healthy lifestyle. In recognition of the fact that life isn't always what we would ideally like it to be, the next section, *Damage Limitation*, is devoted to crisis management. Read on to find out more …

SECTION 3

Life may not always run smoothly, so to keep your new size you need ...

DAMAGE LIMITATION

Have you noticed that as your weight-loss dreams become a reality and exercise a regular part of your life, you start to get a feel-good factor—a kind of rush that actually makes you want to continue eating sensibly and exercising? You actually reach a situation where you are enjoying your healthy lifestyle. As you come to grips with the strategies you learned about in section two, you begin to climb up a self-perpetuating spiral, you look and feel better, you have more energy, which spurs you on to continue.

There you are, looking great, feeling in control, with lots more energy, then BANG! Real life hits you with a genuine crisis or obstacle and your healthy lifestyle goes out the window—just when you felt you were doing so well.

So, you get thrown off your upward spiral and find yourself plunging back to where you started, making unhealthy food choices, having no motivation to exercise and, worst of all, feeling guilty and as if you have failed or let yourself down. You start to feel annoyed with yourself and a bit depressed, which prevents you from taking control of the situation. Eventually, you hit the bottom and if you're lucky, pick yourself up and start again.

THE SPIRAL SCENARIO

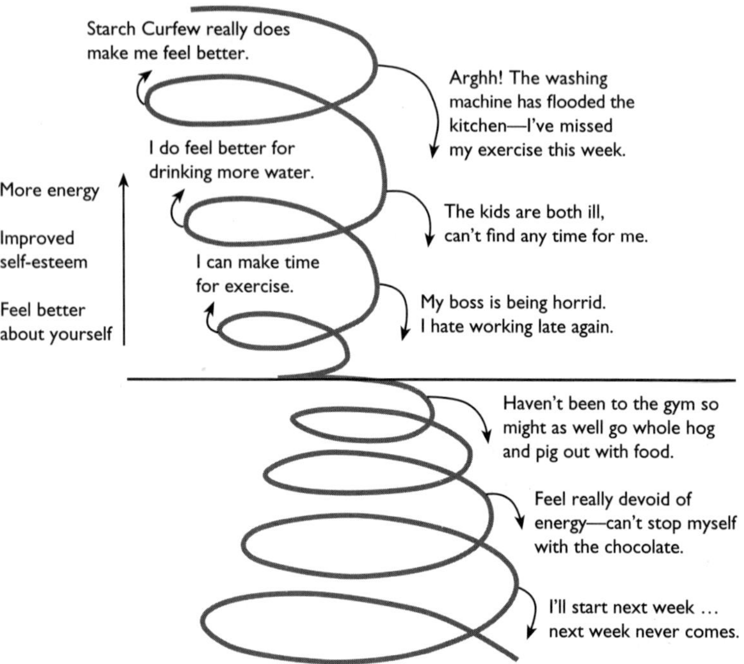

These peaks and troughs of weight gain and weight loss and the accompanying psychological battle we have with ourselves can be damaging not only to our body's health but also to our long-term self-esteem and body image. Studies show that women with low self-esteem and negative body image are less likely to exercise and more likely to practice unhealthy eating behaviors such as fasting and bingeing or using laxatives and diet pills. So how can you avoid being thrown off your upward spiral? It is how you deal with life's rich and varied situations that can really make an impact on your long-term success. So instead of letting such difficulties get the better of you, in this section you'll find a variety of problems and solutions to help you keep on track. I call this Damage Limitation.

WHAT IS DAMAGE LIMITATION?

The key to practicing successful damage limitation is learning how to identify and deal with potentially problematic situations. Sometimes, they are small things—like nibbling the childrens' leftovers—that have just become a habit that's really difficult to break, or maybe a bigger event—like a weekend of partying at a wedding, or a traditional Sunday lunch get-together—has you in a panic. Maybe you are a chocoholic, or stress has you reaching for the candy machine. Whatever it is, we all have a situation where we find self-control difficult, or even impossible, and we often find ourselves ditching all our good intentions. And you know what? That is OK—it is OK to have some chocolate, it is OK to have that splurge—life is about having a good time, after all. But the problem comes when we see one minor hiccup as the end of everything positive we have achieved. Yes, we all get knocked off our spiral every now and then but, instead of slipping all the way down, damage limitation will help you find solutions to the challenges and problems you experience in your life, enabling you to maintain weight loss, an active lifestyle, and a healthy body image. Not all the following situations will present a challenge to you, but there are plenty of solutions, tips, and recipes that you can incorporate into your own damage-limitation strategy.

If you feel that maintaining a healthy diet and finding time to exercise is just too much, you may feel that you can only do one or the other. If you put me on the spot, I'd have to say that being physically active—whether it's through Moving More, More Often, or through Structured Exercise—is the single most important strategy you can adopt and maintain; it directly improves your health, helps boost your self-esteem, and controls your body composition—meaning you will be burning more calories, even in your sleep. What you eat is of the utmost importance too, but if one is going to be temporarily put aside due to other commitments or difficulties, do try to keep up your physical activity.

PROBLEM: THE FAMILY ALL EAT AT DIFFERENT TIMES

Not eating as a family can cultivate some bad eating habits, not just with you but also with the rest of the family. A week-long survey of 289 highschool students by the Childrens' Nutrition Research Center in Dallas revealed youngsters who had dinner with their parents ate lower-fat foods and more fruit and vegetables. Overweight children reported eating at least half of their meals in front of the television. Meanwhile, a Spanish study of 282 teenagers who shared at least five family meals a week, found they suffered less anxiety and depression, regardless of their parents' education level or whether both parents worked outside of the home.

SOLUTION:

DAMAGE LIMITATION

- Make a family dinner date

Check schedules and make a date when you can sit down together for dinner. Mark everyone's calendars and tell them their attendance at dinner is requested. You could even write invites to make it more of a special occasion.

- Bring home healthy, fast food

Try pre-cut, frozen, canned, or microwave-in-the-bag vegetables. Turn up the nutrition on canned soups by adding frozen vegetables and pre-cooked chicken breasts.

- Dig out the slow cooker

Toss in frozen chicken breasts, a bag of frozen carrots, chopped onions, and a jar of low-salt sauce before you leave for work. Your meal will then be ready when you are.

■ Sit down on the run

If you only have time for a quick bite at a fast food outlet (see below) you can still make it a healthy affair. For example, choose grilled chicken with no sauce and remove the skin, or a single burger with lettuce and tomato instead of a triple cheeseburger. Order side salads (hold the dressing) and skip the carbonated drinks, opting instead for low-fat milk, water, or juice. Unfortunately, pizza can be a nutritional minefield, laden with cheese, high-fat meat and oil. The main problem, however, is the size of the helping you're usually given. If you're eating out, share a pizza with a friend and fill up with a side salad. Or ask the restaurant to use half the usual amount of cheese along with a variety of vegetable toppings.

PROBLEM: EATING OUT

Let's get one thing straight—living a healthy, balanced life should be about going out and having a good time. Long-term weight management should not leave you feeling you cannot accept invitations from friends and family or enjoy a meal in a restaurant while you are building your new healthy eating habits. So when your dinner invitation arrives, here are some solutions to help you.

SOLUTION: DAMAGE LIMITATION

■ Operate a starch-free zone

A starch-free zone is a useful strategy to help you keep

your calories balanced when operating the Starch Curfew just isn't possible. Instead of having a Starch Curfew dinner and causing all sorts of complications for your host, have a Starch Curfew lunch instead. This allows you to include some starch with your evening meal without over-indulging.

When eating out at a friend's, I usually go along with whatever they are having rather than causing a fuss. But I do not have such big portions as I used to do, or go back for second helpings. I also skip the bread and stick to just one glass of wine. When eating out in a restaurant, I used to allow myself whatever I wanted—it wasn't until I started the plan and kept track of my eating habits that I realized how often I ate out and acknowledged that I needed to choose more suitable options. While on vacation recently, out of four nights eating in restaurants, I had baked hake, broiled lemon sole, fillet steak, and monkfish. No calorie-laden sauces, deep-frying or desserts for me! Changed times, thanks to the Get a Grip *plan.*
Joan, 63

■ Eat in two acts

This is a useful strategy for those of us who overeat when away from our home territory. Divide the food on your plate in two halves. If you are dining out, you can make an imaginary line. Eat half the food. Stop for 10 minutes and either leave the table, or sip a glass of water until it's empty. If you are still hungry after 10 minutes, finish your meal. If you are not sure, divide the remainder in half and repeat the exercise.

- Order first, drink later

Place your food order before you have your glass of wine. Alcohol loosens your inhibitions, which makes you less careful when ordering. It also makes you feel less satisfied after your meal, resulting in an increased calorie intake over the next 24 hours.

- My usual, please

If you have a favorite restaurant that you visit frequently, decide ahead what you would like to order, basing your choice on the Habit Building principles you learned in Section Two. That way, you won't be tempted when you open the menu. When your resolve is weak, tell someone what you would like to order and visit the bathroom while the order is being taken so your decision can't be shaken.

- Buffet Management

Buffets are the dieter's downfall. An American study recently found that people ate a staggering 44 percent more when they were able to select from a variety of dishes, compared to being offered the same amount of just one dish. So at buffets, try limiting your variety of foods to two per plate, that way you are not over-eating all in one go. Allow yourself to go back as many times as you wish but enjoy the flavors you have on your plate one at a time.

■ Portion Control

Fill your plate with vegetables, salad and lower-calorie foods and then finish off with one or two of the other buffet fillers, remembering to keep a check on portion sizes. Turn to page 166 for a reminder of what a standard portion of some common foods looks like.

■ Prioritize your eating

Once back at your table eat the lowest-calorie foods first (these are generally the vegetables). Then eat the next-lowest-calorie item. Save your highest-calorie item for last. You'll get the taste, but you may just find yourself too full to finish it.

■ Don't starve, eat less

If you know you've got a splurge coming, try eating a little less the day before. Aim to eat 300 calories less, make sure you meet your physical activity targets, and you can enjoy your excesses a little more without feeling guilty. The day after you overeat return to your habit building.

PROBLEM: YOU ARE STRESSED

Stress is a very common trigger for overeating—you either do it to "comfort" yourself from the trials and tribulations of the day, or you do it mindlessly—barely aware that you are eating at all. Just look at how this "mindless nibbling" can impact on your weight-loss efforts …

THE PERILS OF MINDLESS NIBBLING

Food	What it costs in calories	If you did it every day you'd gain ...	If you were able to do it only twice a week you'd save ...
2 teaspoons peanut butter	125	13lb in a year	625 cals
Large handful of salted peanuts	300	31lb in a year	1500 cals
Tablespoon of cake mix	120	12.5lb in a year	600 cals
Matchbox-sized piece of cheese	115	12lb in a year	575 cals
Finishing off kids' 2 sausages	220	23lb in a year	1100 cals
Eating the children's left-over buttered toast	130 a slice	13.5lb in a year	650 cals
Handful of fries	115 (for half a small bag)	12lb in a year	575 cals

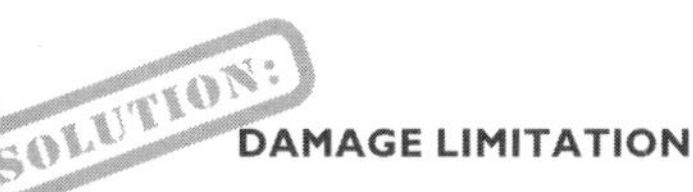

DAMAGE LIMITATION

■ Opt for "eat slow" snacks

Foods that are hard to eat take longer to finish, which gives the brain a chance to register what you have actually put in your stomach. Here are some ideas: a baked apple, a large bowl of air-popped popcorn, a bag of pre-cut carrots with low-fat dip, or an artichoke with low-fat dressing.

■ Move more, more often

Exercise, particularly low-to-moderate intensity aerobic activity, has been shown to reduce stress and anxiety. Refer back to Move More, More Often and Structured Exercise on pages 102 and 116 for ideas on how to inject a little more activity into your life and combat stress.

■ Get the right perspective

Acknowledging that you are in a stressful phase of your life is really important. Now is the time to praise yourself for any healthy activity or strategy you are maintaining, rather than beating yourself up for not doing more. So even if you've failed to operate the Starch Curfew or fit in structured exercise, perhaps you've managed to drink your daily quota of water and walked to the bus stop every day. Be patient with yourself, and practice a positive mantra such as "I am taking care of my body while it sees me through this stressful situation."

■ Raise yourself up the priority list

Get a piece of paper and answer the following questions:
Who is the most important person in your life?
After that person, who is the most important person in your life?

Look at the names you wrote down. Do you see your name? If you do, well done. If you don't, think how many more layers of other "more" important people you would list before you wrote down your own name. If you are the primary homemaker in your family, you will probably be the one person who holds your family unit and everyday activities together. You are the most important person in keeping all the other people in your life happy, healthy and safe—yet unless you start looking after yourself you are not going to keep every other aspect of your life going. You need to raise yourself up the priority list, because unless you start looking after yourself, you are going to feel unhappy, less healthy and more rundown and you are not going to be able to care for those important loved ones. This is one of the hardest things for many women to realize: we need to embrace the fact that taking a little time out for ourselves—for exercise and healthy nutrition—will keep the whole thing moving. Once you understand this and put it into practice you will feel better and you will be able to ride the wave of stress much more successfully.

PROBLEM: ENTERTAINING AND CELEBRATORY MEALS

Whether it is a classic Sunday dinner, Christmas feast, or a dinner party for friends, this type of meal is traditionally when we stock up and enjoy food and drink to excess. And to tell you the truth, this isn't a great problem. While a really excessive Christmas dinner with all the trimmings can add up to a total of nearly 7000 calories, it generally isn't that one day of excess that piles on the pounds, but rather the slow steady accumulation of calories over the whole holiday season, or the action you have taken over the course of the week. Remember, to gain a pound of weight you need to eat an additional 3500 calories a week—so that Christmas dinner should only be adding a couple of pounds. Think about it—if we want to lose a pound, we must try to achieve a calorie burn of 500 calories each day, therefore if we start eating an additional 500 calories a day, week in, week out, the pounds start to pile on and our health is negatively affected.

The physical activity habits that you learned in Habit Building start to become very important at these times. Remember, the weight that you will be in 24 months will not be determined by what you do for the next 24 hours or 24 days but by what you can keep doing for the next 24 months.

I started Joanna's plan a few months before Christmas, two years ago. I lost nearly 15 pounds and I was really pleased. Over that first Christmas I was not very good with my habit building and gained back nine pounds. I was a bit disappointed. Over the next 12 months I continued to lose weight and decrease my body fat. I really got to grips with being consistent with my habits—especially increasing my physical activity levels. Yes, I had a few blips and I certainly was not good the whole time, so I approached the next Christmas with apprehension. When I weighed myself this time, I had only gained three pounds and I certainly ate all the Christmas goodies. Being consistent had worked—it was almost as if my body had got used to dealing with this extra load of calories and instead of saying "I'll store this as fat," I was able to burn it off. **Judith, 53**

SOLUTION:

DAMAGE LIMITATION

■ Operate a starch-free zone

See page 182 to find out how.

If you feel that you'll be selling your guests or family short by making healthier food choices, think again. Not only will you be doing everyone's health a favor, they won't even notice that you're implementing dietary strategies because the food you serve is so delicious! To prove the point, check out the Sunday dinner menu on page 233.

PROBLEM:

YOU CAN'T RESIST CHOCOLATE

WHY DO WE CRAVE CHOCOLATE?

There are times when nothing but chocolate will do. Chocolate cravings can occur because you are feeling lethargic and feel you need a sugar fix to give you an instant energy boost. Look to your lunch and your hydration levels. Check you are eating the right food ratios at lunchtime (see page 157) and increase your intake of slow-release carbohydrates. Cravings can also be psychological—you remember being given chocolate to soothe or reward you as a child and feel that it will make you feel better as an adult, too.

SOLUTION:

DAMAGE LIMITATION FOR CHOCOHOLICS

■ Phone a friend

Before you dive into that tempting family-sized bar of chocolate you bought for company, call a friend and tell her what you plan to do. It will help you weaken your "need" to eat it.

■ Satisfy chocolate urges safely

When only chocolate will do, try these single servings, but don't keep them in the house:

Snack-size chocolate bar

Finger of fudge

Low-calorie hot chocolate drink

Chunks of frozen banana dipped in low-fat chocolate yogurt

Thick and Creamy Chocolate Milk Shake

This recipe will help curb chocolate cravings—the milk provides essential calcium and the volume of the drink stretches your stomach, sending messages to the brain that you are full.

1 package low-fat cocoa instant powder
Ice cubes
Half a banana, cut into chunks and frozen
280ml skimmed milk

Dissolve the cocoa in a little hot water and fill up half the cup with cold water. Place in a blender, add some ice cubes, the frozen banana chunks and skimmed milk and blend for about 60 seconds. Pour into a glass and drink.

> *Joanna's top tip:* **The frozen banana chunks are the vital ingredient here as they really thicken the shake and make you feel you are being very self-indulgent!**

I found this recipe great—it really satisfied my chocolate cravings and I found it very filling and quick to make. I enjoyed it so much I used to have it every evening before I started cooking the family dinner—it really helped me to stop picking as I was preparing the meal.
Pam, 46, a self-confessed chocoholic, lost 14 pounds

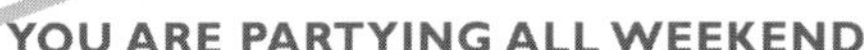

YOU ARE PARTYING ALL WEEKEND

Do you see Monday through Friday lunchtime as your "diet" days and the weekend as the chance to let your hair down, party, and drink and eat what you want? If you are prepared to punish yourself all week to make up for the damage you do at the weekend, you are effectively living the No Air diet (see page vii) from Monday to Friday, week in, week out, and will probably be experiencing frustration at never really seeing the scale shift despite depriving yourself all week. If this sounds like you, and you feel that the only thing to do is stop partying altogether—well, you may be surprised, but I'm actually not going to tell you to do that. Firstly, you need to stop depriving yourself from Monday to Friday and start building in some little actions that mean you can party at the weekend. You'll need to ease back a *bit* but more importantly, you need to stop your erratic eating behavior.

SOLUTION:

DAMAGE LIMITATION

■ The value of consistency

For you to see a change in the size of your body, you need to give each and every microscopic cell in your body a consistent message. Unless you are able to do this, you will not see much of a change in your body. Being consistent does not mean you have to be a goody two-shoes all the time—being consistent means that by building the habits you learned about in Section Two 80 percent of the time, you *will* see a change in your body shape, you *will* have more energy and you can party at the weekends and *not* see the scale go sky high come Monday morning.

And the best thing is, the longer you are able to build healthy habits, the more comfortable your body will become with occasional periods of excess. The abrupt increase in calories will not be laid down as fat and any weight gain will be more easily lost when you get back into your habit building—particularly if you take care to remain as active as possible.

I lost 28 pounds by following Joanna's plan and I kept it off—all my patients were amazed. Even when I went on vacation to Italy for a week and really partied and pigged out on the pasta, I only gained three pounds, and a week after coming back I was back into my habit building and lost those three pounds—this really does work. **Tony, 46**

■ Don't rob Peter to pay Paul

If you know you are heading for a weekend of excess, don't starve yourself all week. Instead eat 300 calories less the day before your partying begins and be sure to fit in a structured exercise session. Then eat 300 calories less the day after your partying has finished. If your body feels up to it, do another structured exercise session, but you may find it more appropriate to hit your step-walking targets. Carry on being consistent through the rest of the week.

■ Double Starch Curfew

If you have a weekend of weddings, parties, or other back-to-back social events, operate a double Starch Curfew zone. Have a starch-free lunch and a Starch Curfew supper. I suggest this because the chances are your fat intake will be higher on these days, pushing up your calorie intake and it will be easier to minimize increased calorie intake, by avoiding starch rather than trying to avoid the fatty foods.

■ Stay hydrated

After a weekend of excess you will feel tired—make sure you do not compound your feelings of tiredness by being dehydrated as well. Remember, drink little and often.

■ Veggie up

Make yourself up a cauldron of vegetable soup to eat before you go out in the evening—this will curb your appetite and line your stomach.

Here's a great recipe for a hearty vegetable soup. If you don't want such a filling meal, look at the smoothie options on page 219.

Hearty Vegetable Soup

Serves 4

It's a good idea to make double and freeze for later.

2 teaspoons olive oil
1 onion, chopped
½ head cabbage, cut into 2-inch pieces
2 carrots, cut into 1-inch pieces
2 celery stalks, cut into 1-inch pieces
1 zucchini, cut into 1-inch pieces
4 small red potatoes (with skin), cut into 1-inch pieces
2⅓ cups fresh mushrooms, sliced
6 tomatoes, peeled, seeded and diced
1⅔ cups chicken stock
fresh chopped basil
1 tablespoon fresh thyme, chopped
½ teaspoon salt
¼ teaspoon freshly ground black pepper

Heat the oil in a large pan, over a medium heat. Add the onion and cabbage and sauté until tender, about 5 minutes. Add the carrots, celery, zucchini, potatoes, and mushrooms and simmer for 5 minutes.

Add the tomatoes, stock, basil, thyme, salt and pepper. Bring to a boil, reduce the heat to low and simmer until the potatoes are tender, about 30 minutes.

Note: If you are practicing the Starch Curfew you can omit the potatoes.

PROBLEM:

CAN'T GET AWAY FROM THE KITCHEN

If you spend a lot of your day in the kitchen, then chances are you are faced with temptation continually. Maybe you clear the remains from your children's plates, nibble on snacks absentmindedly, or just pick throughout the day instead of eating real meals. Or perhaps you are so used to being in the kitchen you find yourself wandering in and out of the fridge with no specific reason at all. Contrary to popular belief, the calories you consume while standing next to the fridge *do* count!

I keep a bowl of fresh fruit salad in the fridge, also small bowl of fruit Jello for times when I want something sweet, or salad bits—cucumber, celery, radishes, or the occasional pickled onion or walnut, for a savory snack. **Vanessa, 55**

SOLUTION:

DAMAGE LIMITATION

- Plate patrol

If you can't resist inhaling the remains off everyone else's plate as you clear away, then allocate someone to clear the table and clear the scraps straight into the garbage can. Then you can continue with your kitchen duties with temptation firmly out of the way.

■ Join in

If you really can't stop yourself from eating their leftovers, have a side salad for your appetizer and then put all the stored-up leftovers on a plate and eat them as your main meal.

■ Role model

Think about it—you are your child's most influential role model. The visual and verbal images you give your children will have a direct impact on how they feel about food. So your actions are really important—making time to sit down with your children is not only important to help you keep your eating habits sensible and healthy but you are also giving them a fundamentally important message, too.

■ Remind yourself

If you snack absentmindedly, wind a colored band-aid or wrap a piece of fabric around your "eating hand" so every time you go to eat, you can see what you're doing. It will help you not to follow through on your impulse to eat, as well as provide insights into the types of "triggers" that have you heading for the cookie jar.

■ Think beyond baking cookies

If you love your time in the kitchen and enjoy giving food as a gift, think beyond cookies and cakes. Try infused vinegars and salsas. Avoid making baked foods that will be really hard to resist nibbling at, so if you volunteer to make something for a charity event or school fair, opt to make the seasoned oils and vinegars rather than the cookies.

■ Never eat on two feet

Resolve never to eat on two feet. If you can't stop nibbling—that's fine, but make sure whatever it is you are going to sample, you sit down to eat and don't wander around. Make this your mantra and you could be surprised at how many calories you save.

■ Kitchen sleep-walking

If you find yourself walking into the kitchen when you really have no need to and raiding the fridge, why not shut that kitchen door once you have completed everything you need to do in there and put a large piece of tape over the door. That way, when you have to go into the kitchen you can make sure you are going in because you need to rather than just for the sake of it.

PROBLEM:

WEEKENDS LET YOU DOWN

You find it easy to be "good all week" but at the weekend, when there's less of a routine, you let it all go.

SOLUTION:

DAMAGE LIMITATION

■ Try the two-meal tool

At weekends, we often have two meals quite close together.

Many of us have breakfast late and then lunch an hour or two later. Both these meals will also tend to be a bit bigger than you would have during the week. Save calories by having just two meals a day at weekends, breakfast and dinner, and opt for a snack in between. See *In Your Mouth in 5 Mins* (page 224) for substantial snacks that are healthy and nutritious.

■ Cook on a full stomach

If you have to bake or prepare for a dinner party, try to do it when you are full, after a meal or in the morning. Your willpower will be higher and you will be less prone to nibble the whole time.

■ Stretch your lunch

If you know you always get hungry in the afternoon, split your lunch into two sittings. Eat half at your normal lunchtime and the remaining half in the afternoon—but make sure you sit down for it rather than eating it at the fridge.

PROBLEM: TIME OF THE MONTH

Many women find that try as they might, they just can't resist those food cravings at the time of the month. Studies show that in the two weeks leading up to your period, your metabolic rate actually increases by about 140 calories. So now you know why you are more hungry and want to eat more food. The problem is that chocolate bar you are craving will, on average, provide 250 calories, so that means an excess of 110 calories already!

SOLUTION:

DAMAGE LIMITATION

- Opt for 100-calorie snacks
- 2 squares of a bar of chocolate
- 2 crackers
- any piece of fruit
- 20 almonds
- 8 dried apricots
- 4oz pot low-fat yogurt and a small banana
- a palmful of sunflower and pumpkin seeds
- 2 rice cakes topped with cottage cheese
- half a small avocado filled with salsa

- Allocate a binge zone

If you really feel you are not going to be able to resist a binge, then define your zone. Allocate yourself a time when you can binge, for example 9–11 p.m., but during that time eat your fill of the lowest-calorie foods possible —try bowls of water-packed fruits like strawberries or melon, or some steamed vegetables. You will be full, but will have more chance to stay within your calorie limit.

- Take time out

When you feel your eating is out of control, you need to

disconnect temporarily from the activity of eating so you can decide whether you want to continue. Remember you are in control, but you need to give yourself some space to realize this. Get up from the table, brush your teeth, or stop and clean a room in the house. Do whatever it takes to give yourself a break. Your brain needs time to register it is full, and studies have shown this takes about 20 minutes from the act of eating to your brain registering that it is full.

■ Switch the taste sensation

You can help stop a binge in its tracks by switching to a completely different food the moment you catch yourself at the point of bingeing. So if you have started to polish off a tub of ice cream, put the tub away and pull out a bag of fruit or carrot sticks. It will give you an opportunity to create some distance from the easy-eating, high-calorie food.

PROBLEM: TRAVELING

Traveling and being away from your normal environment can be a killer: dealing with different time zones, different food choices, perhaps deciphering different food cultures and languages and, of course, being just plain tired. Of course, you don't have to travel abroad to confront the perils of taking time out—just about any kind of trip can interfere with our good intentions.

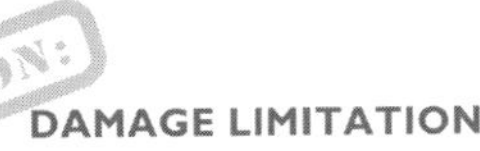

DAMAGE LIMITATION

■ Pre-order your meal

If flying, pre-order a special meal. This is quite easy to do and the airlines are quite happy to do this when asked, except they tend not to make it public knowledge. There is a wide range of special meals you can order—low fat, low calorie, low cholesterol, kosher, vegetarian, to name a few. From my personal experience, different airlines use different criteria to define these different meals. I have found, however, that the veggie option is almost invariably higher in fat than other choices as it is usually based on cheese! So don't pre-order this. So far I have not come across an airline that will specifically prepare you a Starch Curfew dinner—but keep asking, one day they will say yes! Failing that, I'd recommend you request a low-calorie meal. I suggest this rather than the low-fat meal as I have found this often turns out to be a low-cholesterol meal that still has an overall high fat content. The low-calorie options I have had tend to be a better meal all round. And remember to say no to the bread roll and drink plenty of water.

■ Prior protein

Prior to starting out, make sure your last meal has a good balance of protein and starch, so you feel satisfied and motivated as opposed to lethargic. Even athletes traveling around the world to compete use this strategy to minimize the detrimental effects of traveling on their performance.

This pre-flight strategy is also very useful if you are embarking on a long car journey. In this case, you may prefer to just have a smaller protein meal with lots of vegetables and fruit. Remember not to eat too much or your blood sugar levels will rise too quickly and you'll wind up feeling lethargic.

■ Don't "fill'er up"

Resolve not to loiter by the candy counter at the gas station. If you must buy something, grab some chewing gum and a bottle of water or hard candies that take longer to eat, rather than a bag of jelly beans or chocolates.

I found I had really gotten into the habit of not just paying for the gas but also for a car supply of snacks—I used the children as an excuse, and then I found it was me that was devouring them and not the kids! So now I resolve only to buy myself some gum and save the candy for the kids. As soon as I get in the car I start chewing it so I can't be tempted by the kids' jelly babies!
Lucinda, 37

■ Pack your pedometer

You may not feel like exercising as soon as you arrive at your destination, but do try to move your body—resolve to get 4000 steps on that pedometer as soon as possible. It's a great way to explore your destination, and it'll help you get rid of that "traveling fatigue" feeling. If you are on a business trip and your structured exercise sessions are just not going to happen, resolve to get in your daily 10,000 steps—even if it means getting up a little earlier to get them done.

■ Avoid excess snack baggage

If you are at a bar, or are offered nibbles with your pre-flight dinner, say NO—they are laden with salt and calories and will only add to your excess baggage rather than helping you to go first class with your health!

■ Operate the Starch Curfew wherever possible

It works at home and it works just as well when you're away. Take the opportunity to try varieties of fruits and vegetables that aren't available at home, and restrict starchy foods to lunchtimes.

I travel nearly 200 days of the year. I entertain clients for lunch in one country and in another for dinner—my life sounds glamorous but with the weight I was gaining, my appearance certainly wasn't! I had no energy for exercise and the weight was piling on. Once I started operating the Starch Curfew I lost a lot of weight. I found I had more energy and I did not have to feel awkward when ordering in front of clients at a restaurant over a business dinner. No one ever knew I was on a "diet". To me it is not a diet, it is a strategy and, as a businessman, I can really get behind that. The Starch Curfew works! **Richard, 48**

GET A GRIP, HABIT BUILDING OR DAMAGE LIMITATION?

When you picked up this book, you were probably feeling motivated and ready to put your weight-loss plan into action. However, over the weeks of your program there may have been times when your motivation waned a little or life got very hectic and you weren't able to put into practice as many of the habit-building action points as you would have liked. Well, that's life. It's meant to be enjoyed, so let's embrace the things we can do and not beat ourselves up for the things we can't. Every small thing you do matters, so be proud of your efforts. Now that you've read through all the sections of the book, you have probably realized that at some times more than others, you will face challenges and difficulties in maintaining your new healthy habits. It is important to plan ahead and identify when you may experience these difficulties and approach them with the right attitude.

To help you do this, I suggest you identify your weeks by the following categories:

PROGRESSIVE

A progressive week is a week when you feel motivated, you are clear about what you need to do and you are able to put all your tasks in action. You feel confident about being able to fit in your exercise and follow the nutritional guidelines.

HABIT BUILDING

This is when you know it will be a little challenging to get all the tasks completed. Maybe the challenges are due to a deadline you know you have to complete at work and you have to work late, or a member of your family or a friend is unwell and you have to look after them. These are weeks when you may not be able to complete all your tasks, but you can still consolidate your efforts and think about building your healthy lifestyle habits. For example, focus on always drinking your water each day and completing your walks. You are still making progress in these weeks, as habit building is a crucial process not just in realizing your weight-loss goals, but also in keeping the weight off.

DAMAGE LIMITATION

This is when life gets really manic. Maybe you are moving house, changing jobs, going to lots of parties, or the washing machine floods your home ... All of these situations can really throw you off your good intentions. It is quite common for these situations to make you feel like giving up for that week and starting a week later. You may be thinking—I'll forget about this week and start again in earnest next week when things are quieter. This is not a good idea, as next week will come and you will feel as if you have to undo the damage you have done from the previous week. The secret of damage limitation is acknowledging that things may be difficult in the week ahead but planning a few habit-building action points that will help you work toward your goals. These need to be small, achievable things. For example, you don't have time to fit in your walk, but you decide to get up for 60 seconds every hour and do some exercises. You know you won't have time to cook so you check out the diet plan and stock up on some ready-prepared stand-bys such as sushi, soups or prepared fruit salads. This way you will still be feeling positive about your actions and when things calm down, you won't feel as if you have to start again to continue working toward your goals.

As you continue with this program it is a good idea to look ahead and identify whether the coming week will be a Progressive, Habit Building, or Damage Limitation one. We are not always in the ideal situation of being able to do everything right, but the good news is, we don't have to do everything right all the time in order to get—and stay—fit and healthy. So be realistic about what you can achieve, continue to use the skills you've learned in this program and try to devise an effective routine, so you will not just lose the weight, but keep it off.

RECIPES AND RESOURCES

In this section you will find lots of ideas to expand your repertoire of healthy recipes. You can, of course, continue to use the recipes featured in the 14-day *Get a Grip* plan—the recipes featured here are not designed to replace these, simply to give you more choice once you have completed the initial diet and are ready to take up healthy eating permanently. To encourage you to keep up your intake of liquid-based foods I have included a number of ideas for soups and smoothies. You will also find quick and easy snacks and Starch Curfew meals, as well as some recipes for entertaining—including a Sunday dinner menu and some dips and canapés for parties.

SOUPS

Soups are filling and healthy and should definitely be added to the list when you're thinking about what to have for lunch. There's no need to spend ages chopping up vegetables, though. Many of the following soup recipes use quick, convenient ingredients without compromising taste—for instance ready-made soups as a base and packages of ready-prepared vegetables to give added flavor and nutritional value. For a Starch Curfew meal, check that any soup you use as a base doesn't include potatoes, wheat flour, or pasta.

Spicy Corn and Fish Chowder

Serves 2–3

1 carton spicy corn chowder
1 piece (about 10½oz) smoked haddock—use a piece of unsmoked fish if preferred
1⅓ cups skimmed milk
half a head of broccoli, cut into bite-size florets or ¼ cauliflower cut into florets

Info per serving:
Calories: 242.0
Fat: 5.8g
Saturated Fat: 2.5g
Protein: 21.5g
Carbohydrate: 24.4g

Preheat the oven 200°C/400°F.

Put the fish in shallow ovenproof dish and pour the

milk over the fish. Cook in the oven for 10 minutes. Remove from the dish and break the flesh up into bite-size chunks (checking to see there are no bones at the same time).

Microwave the broccoli or cauliflower in a little water for 3 minutes on high. Pour the soup into a pan and heat through. At the last minute, add the smoked haddock and vegetables and stir in well.

Wild Mushroom Soup

Serves 2–3

1 carton wild mushroom soup
light olive oil
3–4 mushrooms, thinly sliced
1 teaspoon freeze-dried parsley or thyme
good handful of bean sprouts

Info per serving:
Calories: 133.0
Fat: 6.8g
Saturated Fat: 3.3g
Protein: 6.6g
Carbohydrate: 11.2g

Gently heat the soup in a saucepan.

Meanwhile, stir-fry the mushrooms in ½ teaspoon of oil on a high heat for 1 minute. Add the herbs and bean sprouts and cook for 30–40 seconds. Divide the heated soup between the bowls and pile the mushrooms and bean sprouts in the center.

Carrot and Cilantro Soup

Serves 2–3

1 carton carrot and cilantro soup
¾cup skimmed milk
1 tablespoon low-fat Greek or natural yogurt
fresh cilantro
freshly ground black pepper

Info per serving:
Calories: 91.0
Fat: 2.70g
Saturated Fat: trace
Protein: 6.0g
Carbohydrate: 10.6g

Empty the soup into a large bowl. Add the milk and chill. Divide the soup between the serving bowls, put a small dollop of yogurt in the center and sprinkle over some fresh cilantro and pepper.

Very Quick Cucumber and Mint Soup

Serves 4

1 cucumber
1⅛ cups low-fat Greek-style yogurt
4 tablespoons skimmed milk
2 garlic cloves, crushed
2 tablespoons chopped fresh mint
2 tablespoons white wine vinegar
salt and freshly ground black pepper
some sprigs of mint for decoration

Info per serving:
Calories: 85.2
Fat: 4.0g
Saturated Fat: 0.1g
Protein: 6.0g
Carbohydrate: 6.7g

Cut the ends off the cucumber and chop roughly. Place in a blender or food processor with the rest of the ingredients and blend until smooth. Check the seasoning and chill until needed. Serve with a sprig of mint floating on top.

Spicy Carrot Soup with a Floating Salad

Serves 4

1 large onion, finely chopped
2 teaspoons minced garlic (available in a tube or jar)
2 teaspoons minced ginger (available in a tube or jar)
1 tablespoon medium curry paste
14-oz can yellow split peas, drained and rinsed
2½ cups carrots, coarsely grated
5¼ cups vegetable stock
1 tablespoon groundnut oil
2 teaspoons onion seeds
1 teaspoon curry paste
11-oz bag stir-fry vegetables (most supermarkets stock them)

Info per serving:
Calories: 332.0
Fat: 2.8g
Saturated Fat: 0.9g
Protein: 19.9g
Carbohydrate: 51.9g

Dry-fry the onion and half the garlic and ginger in a large non-stick pan for 2 minutes—if it sticks add a drop or two of water. Stir in the tablespoon of curry paste and cook for a further minute. Stir in the split peas, carrots, and stock. Bring to a boil and simmer for 25 minutes. Transfer it all to a blender or food processor and blend until smooth. Season well.

Heat the oil in a wok or frying pan and fry the onion seeds until they start to pop. Add the remaining garlic and ginger, the 1 teaspoon of curry paste and the package of vegetables. Stir-fry for 2 minutes. Add salt to taste.

Divide the soup between the serving bowls and pile a little of the salad in the middle of each.

Tom Yum Soup with Mushrooms

Serves 4

This takes a little preparation but it's worth it for a really tasty, very low-cal soup.

2 stalks lemon grass (peel them down to the tender whitish centers)
5¼ cups vegetable stock
2-inch piece fresh root ginger, grated
1 fresh red chili, seeded and finely sliced (wear rubber gloves or wash your hands well afterwards)
¼ teaspoon freshly ground black pepper
2 tablespoons soy sauce
juice of 1 lime
8 button mushrooms, quartered
2 green onions, shredded
small handful of fresh cilantro leaves

Info per serving:
Calories: 48.0
Fat: 0.6g
Saturated Fat: 0.2g
Protein: 3.5g
Carbohydrate: 8.5g

Bash the lemon grass stalks with a rolling pin to crush them and then cut into 1-inch pieces. Put the vegetable stock into a pan and bring it to a boil. Add the crushed lemon grass, cover and simmer on a low heat for 10 minutes. Remove the lemon grass with a slotted spoon and discard.

Add the ginger, chili, black pepper, soy sauce, and lime juice to the stock. Simmer for a further 3 minutes then add the mushrooms. Remove from the heat, cover, and leave for 10 minutes. Serve with green onions and cilantro.

Parsnip Soup with Spinach

Serves 4

1 teaspoon olive oil
1 onion, sliced
1 teaspoon ground cilantro
7 cups parsnips, peeled and coarsely chopped
5¼ cups vegetable stock
salt and freshly ground black pepper

Info per serving:
Calories: 290.0
Fat: 8.0g
Saturated Fat: 1.2g
Protein: 5.4g
Carbohydrate: 48.0g

For the spinach:
1 teaspoon olive oil
2 garlic cloves, sliced
4 cups washed baby spinach

Heat the oil in a large pan and fry the onions and cilantro for 3 minutes until soft and translucent. Add the prepared parsnips and fry gently for 4 minutes.

Pour in the vegetable stock, season and bring to a boil. Cover and simmer on a low heat for about 30 minutes until the parsnips are tender. Cool for a few minutes and transfer to a blender or food processor and blend until smooth. (You may need to do this in batches.) Return the soup to the pan and reheat gently.

Meanwhile, in a frying pan, fry the garlic for a minute and then add the spinach until it just starts to wilt. Spoon the soup into bowls and top with the garlicky spinach.

Quick Curried Corn Soup

Serves 2

1 teaspoon olive oil
1 small onion, chopped
2 garlic cloves, crushed
1 teaspoon curry powder
8oz frozen corn
1⅛ cups dry white wine
2 cups vegetable stock
2 tablespoons low-fat crème fraiche
salt and freshly ground black pepper

Info per serving:
Calories: 265.0
Fat: 10.4g
Saturated Fat: 2.7g
Protein: 5.8g
Carbohydrate: 33.5g

Heat the oil in a large pan and cook the onion, garlic, and curry powder over a low heat for 5 minutes.

Add all the remaining ingredients except the crème fraiche. Bring to a boil and simmer for 10 minutes.

Stir in the crème fraiche and transfer to a blender or food processor and blend until smooth. Taste and adjust seasoning.

Very Easy Pea and Watercress Soup

Serves 4

1 tablespoon olive oil
1 large onion, chopped
2¼ cups vegetable stock
1½ cups frozen peas
3-oz bag watercress

Info per serving:
Calories: 116.0
Fat: 3.9g
Saturated Fat: 0.6g
Protein: 5.8g
Carbohydrate: 15.4g

Heat the oil in the pan, add the onion and cook until soft—3–4 minutes. Pour in the stock and bring to a boil, then lower the heat, add the frozen peas and simmer for 3 minutes.

Pick out and discard the thicker stems of watercress and stir the rest into the soup. Cook for about a minute, transfer to a blender or food processor and blend until almost smooth—there should be a little texture.

SMOOTHIES

Smoothies are great to experiment at home with—when you have complete control over what goes into them. All you need is a blender and you're off. Taste and see is the motto—try loads of different combinations and see what you like. If you or your children have trouble eating enough fruit, smoothies are the perfect answer.

Buy fruit in your local markets, particularly in the summer months when there is so much choice and the prices are lower than in the supermarkets.

Smoothies are great at lunchtime or have them mid-morning or mid-afternoon. For optimum flavor and nutritional value, smoothies are best drunk immediately after making them.

Mango and Peach Smoothie

Makes 2 glasses

1 mango, peeled and flesh coarsely chopped
3 peaches, pitted and coarsely chopped
3 tablespoons low-fat yogurt

Info per serving:
Calories: 185.0
Fat: 0.9g
Saturated Fat: 0.4g
Protein: 3.5g
Carbohydrate: 45.5g

Blend until smooth.

Orange, Pineapple, and Raspberry Fizz

Makes 4 glasses

juice of 3–4 oranges
½ a large pineapple, peeled and coarsely chopped
1 small container of raspberries
1⅛ cups sparkling mineral water

Info per serving:
Calories: 148.0
Fat: 1.0g
Saturated Fat: trace
Protein: 10.0g
Carbohydrate: 22.0g

Blend the fruit until smooth. Strain through a fine plastic sieve and add the sparkling water, stirring in gently.

Apricot, Banana, and Honeydew Melon Nectar

Makes 2–3 glasses

5 ripe apricots, pitted and coarsely chopped
1 banana, peeled and broken up into chunks
half a medium-sized honeydew melon, seeded and cut into chunks

Info per serving:
Calories: 164.0
Fat: 1.0g
Saturated Fat: trace
Protein: 10.0g
Carbohydrate: 26.0g

Place the fruit in a blender and blend until smooth.

Banana, Kiwi, and Orange Nectar

Makes 2 glasses

1 banana, peeled and broken into chunks
1 kiwi, peeled and halved
juice of 3 oranges

Info per serving:
Calories: 141.0
Fat: 0.8g
Saturated Fat: 0.1g
Protein: 2.3g
Carbohydrate: 33.4g

Place the fruit and juice in a blender and blend until smooth.

"IN YOUR MOUTH IN 5 MINS" SNACKS

These are substantial snacks that can also double as light lunches. When hunger attacks, chocolate bars, cookies or just good old toast and butter can seem so much quicker than preparing something nutritious, so these snacks have been designed with speed in mind. All are low calorie and designed to curb your hunger, stimulate your concentration, and boost your blood sugar levels.

It's as easy as pie, all you need to do is choose one item from the "bases" column and one from the "toppings" column. Put them together and away you go!

Bases

2 Ryvita crispbreads
1 slice whole-grain bread
1 slice German rye bread
1 slice sourdough bread
1 medium whole-wheat pitta bread
1 slice mixed-seed bread

Toppings

1. 1oz smoked salmon, 1 tablespoon light cream cheese, ½ chopped green onion plus pickled dill cucumbers
2. 3½oz skinned chicken breasts, 1 teaspoon pesto, 3 shredded lettuce leaves, 1 sliced tomato plus seasoning
3. ½ cup cottage cheese, ½ chopped green onion, 2 slices black forest ham (all fat removed) plus seasoning
4. 2oz low-fat spread, 1 heaped teaspoon creamed horseradish, 3½oz cooked beef slices plus 1 teaspoon sweet onion mustard
5. 2oz low-fat spread, 1 teaspoon horseradish, 2½oz skinned smoked mackerel, 2 shredded lettuce leaves plus chives
6. 4½oz drained tuna in brine, ½ chopped green onion, 1 chopped celery stick plus 1 teaspoon low-cal mayo
7. 1 sliced cooked beetroot, ½ cup low-fat tzatziki (yogurt with cucumber) plus ½ chopped green onion
8. ½ cup reduced-fat hummus, 1 grated carrot plus ½ chopped green onion
9. 3½oz cooked and peeled shrimp, 2 tablespoons natural yogurt, 1 tablespoon mango chutney, ½ teaspoon curry paste, plus 2 shredded lettuce leaves
10. 3½oz drained tuna in brine, ⅔ cup cooked chickpeas, ⅓ chopped red onion plus 1 teaspoon low-cal mayo

EMERGENCY RATION PACKAGE

Keeping a stock of ready-prepared emergency fruit and vegetable rations in a plastic box in the fridge is a great way for avoiding the temptation of unhealthy snacking. They're also good served with lunch.

Try these:

- peeled and quartered carrots
- sticks of celery
- sticks of cucumber
- washed radishes
- small containers of soft fruits and packages of prepared pineapple and melon

You can eat them on their own or team with a healthy dip. Bought dips are great but it's much cheaper and quick to make some yourself. Check out the dip recipes on page 248 for some inspiration.

"ON YOUR PLATE IN 15 MINS" STARCH CURFEW DINNERS

You walk in the door from work, you're tired, hungry and you need to eat. Well, here's the answer—six Starch Curfew dinners that can be on your table in fewer than 15 minutes. Remember to serve your Starch Curfew dinners with unlimited vegetables from the list on page 48.

Quick Glazed Pork Loin Chops

Serves 4

2 tablespoons orange smooth marmalade
1 tablespoon Dijon mustard
½ teaspoon Chinese five-spice powder
4 pork chops

Info per serving:
Calories: 294.0
Fat: 13.0g
Saturated Fat: 5.0g
Protein: 35.3g
Carbohydrate: 6.9g

Preheat the broiler to medium. Mix together the marmalade, mustard, and five-spice powder. Put the chops on the broiler pan and brush the glaze over them. Cook through until meat is no longer pink, about 12–15 minutes, turning over halfway through cooking. Baste with more glaze if needed. This dish is also suitable for barbecuing.

Quick Thai Chicken and Coconut Curry

Serves 4

1–2 tablespoons red or green Thai curry paste
1 lb chicken breasts, cubed
salt and freshly ground black pepper
4 cups broccoli, broken up into florets
¾ cup carton reduced-fat coconut cream
good handful fresh cilantro, roughly chopped

Info per serving:
Calories: 311.8
Fat: 13.9g
Saturated Fat: 9.0g
Protein: 38.4g
Carbohydrate: 8.5g

Mix the curry paste in a saucepan with 2 tablespoons of water. Add the cubed chicken, seasoning and ⅔ cup of water. Bring to a boil, lower the heat and simmer for 12–15 minutes until chicken is tender.

Meanwhile, cook the broccoli in some boiling salted water, drain and add to the chicken along with the coconut cream. Simmer gently for 2–3 minutes. Sprinkle over the cilantro.

Other vegetables can be added, such as sugar snap peas, zucchini or green beans.

Microwave Cod and Cabbage

Serves 4

1 tsp light olive oil
2 slices unsmoked lean bacon, chopped
1 small Savoy cabbage, shredded
⅔ cup vegetable stock
4 cod fillets, skinned
salt and freshly ground black pepper

Info per serving:
Calories: 155.6
Fat: 3.7g
Saturated Fat: 1.0g
Protein: 27.5g
Carbohydrate: 1.6g

Heat the oil in a non-stick frying pan and when it starts to smoke add the bacon, tossing for 3–5 minutes until crisp.

Stir in the cabbage, pour over the stock and cook for a further 3 minutes, stirring all the time until almost tender. Transfer to a microwaveable dish.

Lay the fish on top of the cabbage, and season. Cover with plastic wrap and cook on high in a microwave for 5 minutes until the fish is cooked (the flesh starts to turn opaque).

Cheater's Beef Bourguignon with Chickpeas

Serves 2

1 package Supermarket brand Beef Bourguignon
1 package mixed vegetables
14-oz can chickpeas
5½-oz carton low-fat crème fraiche
1 garlic clove, crushed
salt and freshly ground black pepper

Cook the beef and the vegetables according to the instructions on the packages.

Pour the chickpeas with half the juice from the can into a food processor. Add 1 tablespoon crème fraiche and the crushed garlic and season well. Blend until smooth. Heat the purée in a pan and serve on each plate with the vegetables and the beef stacked on top.

Quick Lamb and Spring Onion Stir-Fry

Serves 4

4 tablespoons soy sauce
4 tablespoons sherry
1 tablespoon sesame oil
2 teaspoons wine vinegar
1 tablespoon groundnut oil
2 garlic cloves, thinly sliced
bunch of green onions, sliced into 2-inch diagonal lengths
1 lb lamb fillet, sliced thinly across the grain

Info per serving:
Calories: 255.0
Fat: 12.6g
Saturated Fat: 3.1g
Protein: 25.8g
Carbohydrate: 5.3g

Mix together the soy sauce, sherry, sesame oil, vinegar and 4 tablespoons of water. On a high flame, heat a wok or frying pan with the oil and add the garlic. After a few seconds, add the lamb and stir-fry for 1–2 minutes until browned. Stir in the soy mixture and allow to bubble briefly. Add the green onions and cook for a few more seconds until they just begin to soften. Serve with some steamed broccoli.

Quick Cod and Tomato Stew

Serves 4

2 chopped onions
1 tsp light olive oil
14-oz can chopped tomatoes
1 tablespoon soy sauce
1 teaspoon fresh or ½ teaspoon freeze-dried thyme
salt and freshly-ground black pepper
skinless cod fillets

Info per serving:
Calories: 185.8
Fat: 2.1g
Saturated Fat: 0.3g
Protein: 20.7g
Carbohydrate: 23.6g

Fry the onions in light olive oil until soft and just turning brown.

Stir in the tomatoes, soy sauce, thyme and seasoning. Bring to a boil, stir well and simmer uncovered until sauce reduces and slightly thickens.

Slide the fish into the pan, cover with a lid and cook gently until the fish is tender, about 5 minutes. Serve with lots of shredded steamed cabbage.

SUMMER SUNDAY ENTERTAINING MENU

It's a beautiful summer's day and you plan to have friends over for dinner on the weekend. Here's a great menu plan that's nutritious, healthy, and follows Starch Curfew.

Serves 4

Beginning with…

Artichokes Vinaigrette

Followed by…

Lemon, Thyme and Garlic-stuffed Roast Chicken with Roasted Vegetables and Wok-fried Greens

And finishing with…

Apple and Blackberry "without the pie" with Greek Yogurt Chantilly

INGREDIENTS FOR THE WHOLE MENU

4 globe artichokes—should be a nice olive green color with no black spots. They are a bit fiddly but well worth it if you like your vegetables!

Vinaigrette—can be bought ready made or make your own using Dijon mustard, white wine vinegar, olive oil, and a crushed garlic clove.

3-lb free-range chicken—you don't need to bother with an over-priced organic bird but free rangers are worth the extra expense.

Bunch of thyme and a bulb of garlic—strip the leaves off half of the thyme sprigs and peel about 10 cloves of garlic but leave them whole.

Half an onion, peeled
1 lemon, cut in half
4 zucchini, halved lengthways and then halved again if thick
1 large eggplant, cut into big chunks
3 red peppers, seeded and cut into chunks
3 red onions, halved and quartered
1 packet fresh asparagus (if in season), cut in half diagonally
1 fennel bulb, trimmed of outer leaves and cut into quarters
2 packages green onions, trimmed but kept whole
light olive oil
1 package greens, trimmed, washed and shredded
dash of Japanese soy sauce
4 Macintosh apples, washed and cored
honey
Brown sugar
small container of blackberries, washed
pot of Greek yogurt, flavored with a little superfine sugar and vanilla extract

Artichokes Vinaigrette

This can be cooked and chilled the day before.

With each artichoke, first cut the stalk off as close to the leaves as possible. Using a pair of scissors, snip the pointed bit off each leaf, working from top to bottom. Pull off the reedy-looking leaves from the base and then give the artichokes a good rinse in cold water. Cook in lots of boiling salted water (to prevent discoloration, don't use an iron or aluminum pan) with a little drop of vinegar. Cook them with the lid on, on a medium heat, for about 30–50 minutes, depending on the size. They are cooked when the leaves come out when tugged gently. Put them in a colander upside down to drain them well and cover and chill when cool.

To serve, place each cooled artichoke on a big plate and season with flaky salt and pepper. Drizzle vinaigrette over each one and have some in a pot if extra is needed. To eat them, pull off the leaves individually and, with your teeth, scrape off the creamy flesh from the bottom of each leaf. When the leaves become thin, diaphanous and reedy, pull them all off and discard. Gently, with a knife, scrape off and discard the hairy choke protecting the heart. Keep a bowl of warm water with a lemon slice to wash your fingers at the table.

Lemon, Thyme and Garlic Roast Chicken

Preheat oven to 180°C/350°F.

First pull out any unwanted bits of fat clinging to the inside of the chicken.

Loosen the skin covering the breast meat carefully with your fingers, trying hard not to pierce the skin.

Crush 5 cloves of garlic and mix them in a bowl with a handful of thyme leaves and 2 teaspoons of salt. Gently push the garlic herb paste in between the flesh and the skin as far and as evenly as possible. Put the remaining whole garlic cloves inside the cavity of the bird along with the thyme sprigs, half a lemon and the half onion. Place the bird in a roasting pan, squeeze over the juice from the remaining lemon half and season well, inside and out, with sea salt and ground black pepper.

Put the chicken in the oven on the middle shelf and roast for about 1 hour, until the juices run clear when the flesh is pierced. Remove the chicken to a serving plate, pour off the fat from the roasting tin and discard. Loosen the juices with a little water or stock if preferred over a low flame for a couple of minutes.

Roasted Vegetables

About 15 minutes after the chicken goes in the oven, the vegetables can go in, on the top shelf. Place the prepared vegetables, except the asparagus (they take less time to cook) in a roasting tray, making sure the onion in particular is evenly distributed in the tin. Drizzle some olive oil over in a thin trickle. Season well and make sure they are all well coated. Check them every 15 minutes, turning them and giving the pan a good shake to loosen any vegetables sticking to the bottom. They will be ready when they turn a light caramel color and are cooked through—about 45 minutes, depending on the intensity of the oven. The asparagus can either be added to the rest of the vegetables with 20 minutes to go, or can be cooked separately using the same method.

If you want to use root vegetables instead, carrots, onions, leeks and parsnips are a good combination—cooked using exactly the same method and, as long as they are all cut into roughly the same-size chunks, taking about the same amount of time.

Wok-fried Greens

Heat a wok until smoking and add 1 teaspoon of olive oil, swilling it around. Add the shredded greens and keep them moving around the wok by stirring all the time. Add about a tablespoon of soy sauce, coating the leaves as much as possible. When the greens have just a little bite to them and have reduced and wilted down a bit, they are ready to serve.

Serve some greens piled into the center of the plate. On top, lay some roasted vegetables, making sure everybody gets a good even mix. Lay the chicken on top and drizzle some of the pan juices over the top.

Apple and Blackberry "without the pie" with Greek Yogurt Chantilly

Preheat the oven to 180°C/350°F.

Place the cored apples into a small roasting pan. Add 2 tablespoons water to the base of the tin. Put some brown sugar into a bowl and roll the still-wet blackberries into the sugar to get a good coating. Push as many sugared blackberries as possible down into the center of each apple. When all four apples are prepared, drizzle some honey over each and put them on the middle shelf, once the chicken has come out. Roast the apples for 30–40 minutes, depending on their size.

Serve warm or cold with a good dollop of the sweetened and flavored Greek yogurt on the side.

FISH OPTION MAIN COURSE

Italian Cod (or monkfish) with Garlic Tomatoes

Serves 4

2 unpeeled garlic cloves
1 tablespoon olive oil
⅔ cup black olives
5½ cups tomatoes, preferably plum—keep them whole with stalks
2 red chilies, seeded and roughly chopped
3 tablespoons fresh pesto
2 boneless, skinless cod fillets or monkfish tails, approximately 1 lb each in weight
grated rind of 1 lemon
12 slices of prosciutto or Serrano ham—fat removed

Info per serving:
Calories: 392.0
Fat: 12.0g
Saturated Fat: 3.6g
Protein: 50.0g
Carbohydrate: 14.9g

Preheat the oven to 200°C/400°F.

Put 2 tablespoons of oil in a roasting pan with the garlic and roast for 15 minutes. Add the tomatoes, olives and chilies to the pan, mixing them in with the oil, and add seasoning.

Spread the pesto over one side of a cod fillet and sprinkle on some lemon juice and seasoning. Lay the other cod fillet on top and loosely wrap the ham slices around the fish, tucking in the edges on either side. Lightly drizzle with olive oil and put the cod on a broiling rack over the pan. Roast the fish for 20 minutes, when the fish should be cooked and the tomatoes starting to break up.

Transfer the fish to a serving plate. Mash the two garlic cloves into the pan juices and throw away the tough outer skins. Serve the fish with the pan juices drizzled over the top. Serve with sautéed zucchini and a green salad.

VEGETARIAN OPTION MAIN COURSE

Baked Eggplant and Fennel with Shallots

This recipe is suitable for vegans if the Parmesan is omitted.

Serves 6

2 large garlic cloves, crushed
2 tablespoons sun-dried tomato paste
6 tablespoons olive oil
1 tablespoon balsamic vinegar
1 tablespoon lemon juice
3 fennel bulbs
1 large eggplant
12 shallots
14-oz can chickpeas, drained
1¼ cups freshly grated Parmesan
1 bunch green onions, sliced diagonally in ¼-inch slices
Coarsely ground black pepper

Info per serving:
Calories: 325.2
Fat: 19.4g
Saturated Fat: 4.3g
Protein: 11.1g
Carbohydrate: 29.0g

Preheat oven to 200°C/400°F.

Into a screwtop jar put the crushed garlic, tomato paste, 2 tablespoons olive oil, the vinegar, lemon juice and black pepper. Give it a good shake.

Top and tail the fennel. Keep back the feathery leaves for later and discard any blemished outer leaves. Slice thinly lengthways and put into a bowl. Top and tail the eggplant. Halve lengthways and cut into chunks. Peel and quarter the shallots and add to the fennel and eggplant, along with the chickpeas. Add the garlic mixture and mix into the vegetables thoroughly.

Put the vegetables into a roasting tin and cook for 30 minutes. Sprinkle with the Parmesan and cook for a further 10 minutes until melted and golden.

Roughly chop the reserved feathery fennel and scatter over the vegetables. Drizzle over the remaining olive oil before serving.

CANAPÉS AND HEALTHY PARTY DIPS

Smoked Salmon Rounds

Makes around 18

6 slices pumpernickel or German rye bread
1½ cups low-fat cream cheese
chives, snipped into ⅕ inch using scissors
10oz smoked salmon
red spring onions, sliced very thinly

Info per serving:
Calories: 65.9
Fat: 1.8g
Saturated Fat: 0.2g
Protein: 6.2g
Carbohydrate: 6.0g

Using a round 2-inch diameter crinkle-edged pastry cutter, cut out rounds of bread from each slice—if you're lucky, you may get 4 per slice.

Mix together the cream cheese and as many chives as you wish to use. If it is a little thick, loosen the cheese with a drop of skimmed milk, but only a drop at a time!

Put the cheese into a small plastic bag and seal the top. Make a little snip in one corner and you have an instant piping bag. Pipe rosettes of cream cheese onto each round—it gets easier with practice!

Cut the smoked salmon into ribbons and drape a couple over the cream cheese. Separate the onion slices into individual rings and balance 3 over the salmon. Enjoy!

Tricolor Skewers

Makes about 24

1 pot 7-oz baby mozzarella balls, each one cut in half
1 packet basil leaves
1 small container baby plum tomatoes or small cherry tomatoes, sliced lengthways
¼ cup pesto sauce
light olive oil
salt and freshly ground black pepper
wooden skewers

Info per serving:
Calories: 44.7
Fat: 3.6g
Saturated Fat: 1.3g
Protein: 1.9g
Carbohydrate: 1.4g

Skewer a half-mozzarella ball. Fold a single basil leaf in half and skewer that on top of the cheese. Then spear the tomato lengthways so the three are at the end of the skewer.

In a bowl mix some pesto with some olive oil to loosen it to almost a pouring consistency. When you have completed all the sticks and just before serving, season them. Serve with the bowl of the pesto nearby for dipping.

SKEWERED MEAT, CHICKEN, AND FISH

Wooden skewers are great for all sorts of bite-size food for parties.

Using any number of bought marinades, marinate some chicken breasts, beef fillet or fish (tuna, swordfish or monkfish are ideal). Cut into bite-size chunks about 1-inch, skewer the meat onto the sticks and broil on a medium heat for a matter of minutes, turning and watching them closely so they don't burn. Pre-soaking the sticks in water for a couple of hours stops them from burning under the broiler. Buy a ready-made salsa as a dip for them.

Snowpeas and Shrimp Skewers

Makes 20

Info per serving:
Calories: 23.4
Fat: 0.3g
Saturated Fat: 0.1g
Protein: 4.8g
Carbohydrate: 0.2g

20 snowpeas, boiled for 1 minute then plunged into cold water
20 large cooked shrimps
small jar of mayonnaise
½ lemon, juiced
wooden skewers

Pat dry the snowpeas so everything is to hand and ready. Hold the shrimp in a "c" shape. Skewer the bottom of the "c". Then take a snowpea and, with the skewer, spear a third of the way from underneath to top. Spear the top of the "c" shrimp, then spear just over halfway up the snowpea from the top so the tip of the skewer is hidden behind the vegetable. It will all make perfect sense once you start spearing! Add the lemon juice to the mayonnaise and offer to your non-dieting guests as a dip with their shrimp.

FRUIT KEBABS

Use shorter skewers for making fruit kebabs. Steer clear from spearing soft berries such as blackberries or raspberries. Have a chocolate dip at the ready for speared strawberries (again for those nasty non-dieters!). Finish off the skewer with a firm fruit like a grape speared lengthways.

DIPS

All dips should be served with really fresh crudités: peeled and halved celery sticks, peeled carrot sticks, unpeeled seeded cucumber, washed "breakfast" radishes, baby tomatoes, broccoli and cauliflower florets, and fennel—trimmed and cut into curvy batons.

Red Pepper Hummus

Makes about 1½ cups hummus

1 seeded and roughly chopped red pepper
1 large garlic clove
14-oz can chickpeas, drained
2 tablespoons light olive oil
1 tablespoon lemon juice
a dash of Tabasco or other "hot" sauce
salt and freshly ground black pepper

Place the ingredients in a food processor and process until reasonably smooth. Season to taste and chill until needed.

Avocado, Feta Cheese, and Tomato

1 large avocado
5-oz carton low-fat spread
2 green onions, finely chopped
½ cup crumbled feta
1 large ripe tomato, seeded and chopped
salt and freshly ground black pepper
Tabasco (optional)

Mash the avocado into the low-fat spread. Stir in the onions, feta and tomato and season with salt and pepper and Tabasco.

Yogurt, Cilantro, and Chutney

6 tablespoons mango chutney
small handful of fresh cilantro, chopped
4 green onions, chopped
juice of 2 limes
¾ cup light cream cheese or low-fat spread
½ cup Greek low-fat yogurt
½ cup low-fat bio yogurt
½ teaspoon curry powder
½ teaspoon turmeric
salt and freshly ground black pepper
Tabasco

Blend everything bar the seasoning in a food processor/ blender. Season to taste and chill for at least 30 minutes.

By leaving out the curry powder and adding the same amount of Thai sweet chili sauce in place of mango chutney, this Indian-style dip becomes a Thai-style dip!

Sun-dried Tomato and Cannellini Bean

14-oz can cannellini beans, drained
8 sun-dried tomatoes in oil, well drained
1 clove garlic, crushed
1 tablespoons light olive oil
2 tablespoons red wine vinegar
½ cup water
salt and freshly ground black pepper

Blend everything except the seasoning in a food processor or blender. If the dip is too thick, add a tablespoon of water at a time for the desired consistency. Season well and chill for at least 30 minutes.

Baby Meringues

Makes 20

These are great "finger desserts" to round off your buffet or barbecue.

2 egg whites
1¼ cups superfine sugar
½ teaspoon vanilla extract

Info per serving:
Calories: 27.0
Fat: 0.0g
Saturated Fat: 0.0g
Protein: 2.3g
Carbohydrate: 5.0g

Preheat the oven to 180°C/350°F. Whip the egg whites in a clean, grease-free bowl until they are stiff and you are brave enough to turn the bowl upside down! Add one spoon of sugar at a time and whisk into the egg white. When all the sugar has been added, the egg whites will be stiff and glossy. Fold the vanilla in with a rubber spatula.

Using two teaspoons, put spoonfuls of mixture onto a greased baking tray at 1-inch intervals. Before putting in the oven, make an indent in each meringue using the back of a teaspoon. Bake for 5 minutes and turn down the oven to 120°C/225°F for 20 minutes. Cool them down completely before removing from the tray.

Fill the meringues with sweetened Greek yogurt with a little whipped cream added and top with fruit:

for example, half a kiwi slice, a raspberry and a few passion fruit seeds or just raspberries and a sprig of mint. Dust with some confectioner's sugar and serve.